Ease and Skill

Marcus James has been an Alexander Technique teacher for over twenty years. He is also a psychotherapist, working with both talk-based and embodied modalities. His therapeutic work incorporates contemporary person-centred, neo-Reichian and somatically informed trauma work. He teaches a therapeutic group dance practice called Dance of Awareness.

Marcus worked for many years as a craftsperson, producing bespoke handmade furniture in a contemporary Arts and Crafts style. He writes poetry and owns a small poetry press.

Ease and Skill

A User's Guide to the Self

Marcus James

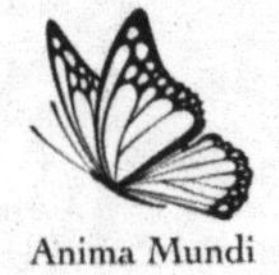

Anima Mundi

Anima Mundi

Published by Anima Mundi

First Edition, 2024
International (non UK) version

Disclaimers

In order to protect the privacy of individuals mentioned,
some identifying details and characteristics have
been changed or anonymised.

The information provided in this book is for educational and infor-
mational purposes only and is not intended as medical advice. The
content is not a substitute for professional medical advice, diagnosis,
or treatment. Always seek the advice of your physician or other
qualified health provider with any questions you may have regarding
a medical condition. Never disregard professional medical advice or
delay in seeking it because of something you have read in this book.

ISBN 978-1-0686869-1-7

For my Students

Familiar acts are beautiful through love.
Percy Bysshe Shelley, Prometheus Unbound

Contents

List of Illustrations vii

Preface xi

Note on Sources xix

Introduction xxi

Part One: Foundations

1. Discomfort and Ease 3

2. Three Views of the Self.. 13

3. Blood Flow and Breathing 18

4. Primitive Emotional Responses.................................. 25

5. Sensing and Attention.. 31

6. Stabilisation.. 38

7. Support... 44

8. Balance 58

9. Movement 65

Part Two: Fundamentals of Skill

10. The Adaptable Self 71

11. Action Sequences and Habits................................... 80

12. Circling the Problem 86

Part Three: The Skilful Self

13. Being and Doing 91

14. Seven Qualities of Ease 94

15. Four Characteristics of Skilful Action 108

16. Paradise Lost 119

17. Unreliable Sensory Appreciation 132

18. The Tangled Thread 136

Part Four: Coming Home

19. Towards Wholeness 141
20. Pausing to Find Ease 155
21. Difficulties with Ease 160
22. Not Doing 165
23. Not-This-Not-That 172
24. Ease and Movement 180
25. Exploring Skilful Action 186
26. Using the Floor 194
27. Towards Complexity 199
28. Energetic Release 205

Part Five: Deepening The Practice

29. Contact, Attunement and Expression 211
30. Trauma 223
31. Emotional Blocks 227
32. The Road Ahead 239

Appendices

A. Note For Alexander Teachers 247
B. When the Right Thing *Can't* Do Itself 255
C. Regulating Anxiety States 258
D. Further Reading 264

List of Illustrations

Fig. 1. The Breathing Mechanism...................................21

Fig. 2. The Bucket Handle Movement (front view)......22

Fig. 3. The Pump Handle Movement (side view).........23

Fig. 4. Axial and Appendicular Skeletons......................45

Fig. 5. Parts of the Spine 47

Fig. 6. The Head–Neck Joint 48

Fig. 7. Superficial Muscles of the Torso.......................50

Fig. 8. Intermediate Muscles of the Torso 50

Fig. 9. Deep Muscles of the Spine and Back 50

Fig. 10. Bones of the Arms and Legs 52

Fig. 11. Muscles of the Shoulder Blades.......................53

Fig. 12. Movements of the Shoulder Blades..................54

Fig. 13. Tendency to Fall Forwards..............................56

Fig. 14. Support From the Back 56

Fig. 15. The Base of Support..59

Acknowledgements

I'm grateful to the worldwide community of Alexander Technique teachers who, for almost a century, have been tenaciously and generously thinking about, experimenting with and sharing this work.

Thank you to Bill Kinghorn, Lena Schibel-Mason and Tim Brown: 'Better than a thousand days of diligent study is one day with a great teacher.'

Thanks also to Maggie Rakusen for her persistence in encouraging me to join her Alexander teacher training course, and to her and Mark Tolson for doing all that was needed to keep it afloat; to Barbara Allen-Williams for encouragement, skilful midwifing and the use of her annexe; to Kate Jones, for listening; to Jean Fischer, Bridget Woodward, Rosie Ferguson, Karen Bali, Julia Brammer, Alison Lee, Tony Donaghy and Safia Minney for reading the manuscript at various stages and making invaluable suggestions for improvement; to Tess Jolly for her skilled and sensitive copyediting of the text; and to Catherine Bone for stepping in at short notice to produce the illustrations.

To my mother, Jane, for her unfailing support.

To Safia, for her love and for sharing the journey.

Preface

This book draws together many threads, but I can trace its origin back to a single hour of my life. I was at music college and in love with the piano—and particularly jazz—with all the enthusiasm of a young man discovering something for the first time that he cared about enough to give himself to completely. When I arrived I was assigned a piano teacher from among several excellent ones at the college, but I wanted to learn with Bill. Bill was a sort of Yoda character. His lectures were eye-opening because they went so much deeper and wider than anything I'd experienced before. Bill skated lightly over the 'what to do' and instead went straight for the depths of 'how things work'—the underlying patterns and the way that disparate things connect. Most jazz teachers don't spend much time on Schenkerian analysis or Schoenberg's structural functions or the teachings of Krishnamurti. Bill did. And not only that but he played the piano like the ghost of Bill Evans, which at that time was right where I was coming from.

So I wanted to learn piano with Bill, and I begged and whined and generally made a nuisance of myself until I was allowed to. I remember turning up for the first lesson rather agog. I think I was maybe a little proud of my playing and what I felt I'd achieved so far. Bill suggested I play something for him. I placed my hands on the keys and played the first three chords of a piece I'd been working on.

'Stop,' said Bill.

That was as far into the piece as we got that lesson. One bar. Over the next hour he took everything I thought I knew about the piano and turned it inside out—and not in a superficial 'do it like this, not like that' kind of way. Instead, he was pointing out that my whole approach to the instrument—how I thought about it, how I was going about learning it, even my understanding of how the machine worked—was quite simply wrong. There was no 'Not bad, let's improve this or that' from Bill. It was 'What you're up to is fundamentally wrong-headed and won't lead to the sort of sparkling, living, breathing playing that you want to achieve. Ever.'

I left feeling rather shattered.

You might think that this would be a dispiriting experience, but it was not: it was like a door opening onto a new world. I realised that the great players I admired weren't just further down the road than me—they were on a different road altogether! I realised that just carrying on, trying to hone what I was already doing and make it better little by little wouldn't get me where I wanted to go. What I needed more than anything was to *unlearn* what I knew so that there was space for some new magic to happen. And I was ready to do it. I wanted to be on that road. The real road.

I unlearned a lot with Bill over the next couple of years. For example, I unlearned my habit of prodding and pushing my fingers into the keybed. You mustn't force your fingers into the piano because it's a waste of energy and jams you up. Skilful piano-playing often feels more like pulling the notes *out* of the instrument (it's a curious thing: if you were here, I'd love to show you). The moment the hammer is on its way to the string—which happens even before the key is fully depressed—all the energy you continue to put into the key has no effect whatsoever. Not only is it wasted but it's working *against* you.

And I started to unlearn the way I held my torso and legs and arms rigidly, using them as nothing more than a fixture to waggle my fingers from. I discovered that by allowing *all* of me to move, breathe and respond to the feeling of the music, I could unlock the musical sense inside me and allow it to flow, and that the little levers of the fingers can be regulated and nested within bigger ones, the forearms, upper arms and torso all working together as one.[*]

And then, putting the pieces back together, I started to discover what it means to *really* learn—to stop hammering away at nothing. We all do that sometimes, I think. Bang on and on with something hoping it'll get better in the end. But Bill encouraged me to let go of these habitual ways of going about things and to get inside how things actually work—to pause long enough to allow a space in which understanding has a chance to arise rather than endlessly repeating something ugly in the hope that it will somehow stop being so. What a blessing to meet a teacher like that!

Around this time, like many musicians, I started to get involved with the Alexander Technique. How can I talk about this work and the effect it has had on my life? In case you don't know, the Alexander Technique helps to promote well-being through a deep reorganisation of habits of awareness, action, posture, movement and balance. Most of us modern humans tend to approach the things we do

---

[*] Bill was influenced in his approach by the American piano teacher Abby Whiteside.

with a lot more mental and physical tension than we need to. Rather than being graceful, open and free, as we evolved to be, we often end up being rather stiff, held and uncomfortable. This puts a lot of stress and strain on our bodies and prevents us from accessing our full potential for skilled activity. In time, all that stress and strain may even result in injury or chronic pain of one sort or another.

The Alexander Technique can help us to access the innate potential for lightness, ease and skilfulness which is our birthright, but which easily gets lost under the pressures of a contemporary way of life that is very different from the one our bodies and minds evolved to expect. It was developed early in the twentieth century by an Australian man called Frederick Matthias Alexander (1869–1955). Many others have followed in his footsteps—probed, questioned, contradicted, cherished and explored further from the seed he planted. I love it. It's one of the most important and transformative things I have done in my life. Perhaps *the* most important. Much of this book is based on the things I've discovered in exploring it.

I loved the Alexander Technique so much I decided to train to teach it myself. For three years I went each morning to a room by a green square in a town in the North of England. Three years during which, in a concrete but very gentle way, I felt myself physically changing. I discovered, for example, that I had a back and a spine, and the true extent of them, and what it means for them to be experienced as a whole and how that gives a sense of greater security—not only to the body but to one's entire sense of oneself. I found that we can release into movement rather than hold on protectively to ourselves. And I discovered (or at least *began* to discover) that we can allow ourselves to be effortlessly supported by our own neuromuscular system and to flow, whether in something as simple as walking across the room or getting up out of a chair, or as complex as playing the piano.

And so, in time, I began to teach. But after a while I started to wonder why some people found it relatively easy to let go of unhelpful patterns of movement and muscular tension, while others would really struggle with it and change very slowly or not at all. And I became curious about the limits of what I was doing, and about the emotional and physical parts of people that didn't quite seem to be touched by the work—or that perhaps even became a little *more* set and rigid even when there was so much positive change in other ways.

Looking for answers, I turned to the world of psychotherapy. Human societies have come a long way in a short time from their origins as small hunter-gatherer tribes surrounded by nature. In exploring how this may affect us, I was drawn to certain embodied psychotherapies and particularly to the work of Wilhelm Reich.* Reich believed that there are stages of emotional and physical development we all go through in the earliest years of our lives, that these stages may be disrupted in predictable ways, and that when this happens it has fairly predictable impacts on how we tend to respond to the challenges life throws at us. According to Reich, these impacts also have a direct correlation with how we live in our bodies, on how and where we hold muscular tension, and hence on our habitual postures, ways of moving and of interacting with others.

---

*Reich had a very direct approach, often using forceful manipulation to release muscular blocks. Some of his more recent followers have developed gentler, more process-oriented ways of working. It is this neo-Reichian approach that has most influenced this book.

Over the years, many of these ideas have enriched my work as an Alexander Technique teacher, together with insights from trauma-focused therapeutic approaches such as those that have developed from polyvagal theory and the work of Babette Rothschild and Peter Levine.

Throughout this journey, life has taken twists and turns which have sometimes surprised me. Woodworking, which had been a hobby, became a passion. I found myself making and selling fine furniture. Music receded. I trained as a psychotherapist and learned to teach a therapeutic dance practice. A love of reading poetry grew into a love of writing it. So much richness and possibility that grew from the Alexander Technique and those early lessons with Bill which gave me a sense I could take ease into new activities and the confidence to give them a go.

So this book brings together three main threads: the Alexander Technique and all that it is, an interest in gently healing and transforming the unhelpful emotional patterning that many of us carry to a greater or lesser extent, and a lifelong passion for learning new skills and helping myself and others to do the activities we love as well as we are able. It's a book about how we can travel hopefully onwards into the future, with renewed resources, artistry and skill. And at the same time it's a book about coming home—finding our way back to the heart of who we are and of who we were born to be.

Note on Sources

This book draws on shared bodies of knowledge and understanding to which numerous people have contributed. While wanting to acknowledge this, I'm also aware that most of my readers will be best served by a text they can trust well enough, that is helpful and flows naturally and freely, and that isn't any harder work than it needs to be. I've therefore chosen not to interrupt the text with references or attempts to justify what I'm saying as we go along. For those who want to dig deeper, there's information about the origins of the main ideas in Appendix A, and suggestions for further reading in Appendix D.

Introduction

Imagine if there could be a sense of ease in whatever you did—whether in sport, dancing, music, or perhaps just in getting up from a chair, walking the dog or going for a bike ride or run on a summer's evening. How would it be to be able to touch a sense of gracefulness in yourself and your activities so that the daily business of living was experienced as light, gentle and free? What if the simple things—to stand, walk, gesture, even just to breathe— became a source of potential wonder and delight? What if enjoyment of the sheer physicality of being human, of being *embodied*, was a way both into better health and perhaps, in time, into an appreciation of a few deeper truths about life and the human condition?

In this book, I'm going to suggest that one path towards such a way of being lies in paying attention to both the way that we *are* and the way that we *do* things. Not just the overtly skilled activities we take part in—the arts, or sport, or work—but also the everyday, ordinary things: the way we go about moving, standing, walking and carrying ourselves in movement and at rest.

I wonder if this sounds a little far-fetched for many of us, caught on the wheel of adult life, responsibility, caring for others or, for some, even basic survival. Perhaps it even sounds a little selfish. In England, where I live, we often seem to have the idea that thinking about ourselves and our wants and needs is a little self-indulgent. One biscuit is quite enough.

Well, here I'm inviting you to take not just one but a whole handful—a handful of self-care, self-regard and pure enjoyment and interest in yourself, in what and who you are as a thinking, breathing, embodied human, and in how you can become more fully, expressively, openly *you*. I'm going to offer ways of looking at things that can help you take greater responsibility for many aspects of your life and which may, along the way, help to resolve some common physical and emotional problems caused by moving and being in the world in unnecessarily stressed, tense, collapsed or unbalanced ways. I'm offering to take you on a rich journey of self-discovery and change.

Is that a selfish journey? Perhaps. Self-indulgent? Undoubtedly. And yet who among us would not be pleased to have a friend, partner, parent or child who was happier, had more energy to share, a greater sense of presence, and less pain and stuckness in their life? We're all works in progress, and though we owe it to ourselves more than anyone, we also owe it to each other to aspire to be as well we can be.

How to Use This Book

Perhaps you're new to the Alexander Technique. Maybe this is the first time you've ever heard of it. Or perhaps you've had a few, or even many Alexander lessons and are now wanting to think about it more widely or from a different point of view. Maybe you've glimpsed possibilities in the work but are still wondering how to integrate it more fully into your life and make it your own. Whatever the case, this book is for you. If you're a newcomer, it will give you a coherent, contemporary approach to the transformative ideas that F.M. Alexander formulated which is broadly in line with current understandings of how the brain and body work. And if you're already involved with the Technique, it may give you some fresh perspectives, offering ways of approaching things that you may find interesting and helpful.[*]

In the first part of the book I'm going to be offering quite a lot of factual information about your mind, body and emotions, and how they interact to produce either ease and skilfulness or discomfort, awkwardness and stress. If this material is new to you, I suggest you resist the temptation to rush ahead to the more practical, 'how to make things better' part that comes towards the end of the book and instead take some time to absorb and understand the information in the first part. This will be helpful, because it's difficult to bring about positive change in a complex system such as ourselves if we don't understand how that system works.

And yet I'm also very aware of the limits of this kind of technical, factual information. It's essential, but it's not enough. We aren't *just* a set of scientific and mechanical principles, and we're more than *just* a system. We're conscious beings having living, breathing experiences which can't be fully reduced to words or adequately captured and described in technical terms.

Think about skiing down a snowy mountainside. A skiing instructor could give you some useful verbal instructions on how to go about it—what posture to adopt, various ways to stop and turn and so on. Likewise, a scientist could tell you a lot about things that *go on* when you're

---

[*] If you want to know more about where the approach outlined in this book comes from, there is information about the lineage of some of the main ideas in Appendix A.

skiing such as momentum, inertia and friction, and how muscles work together to move and support the body. But to really know skiing, you would have to put the book down and go out and do it.

When you got back, you would probably not—unless you were a serious competitive skier—talk about the experience in scientific or technical terms at all. Instead you'd most likely want to communicate, rather breathlessly, the *qualities* of the experience—the excitement, the sense of freedom, the nervous anticipation, the swoosh of the skis over the tightly packed snow and the beauty of the mountains. And you'd also now have a tangible, lived *sense* of it—the *way* you need to lean into corners, the *particular* balance of forces needed to stay upright or to push off at the top of a run, and the sense of using your arms and poles to balance. Certainly you need to know what you're doing in explicit terms to be able to ski, but you also need to be familiar with the tacit aspects of the experience which can't be fully expressed in words.

In this book, then, we're going to have to look at things from more than one point of view, and sometimes I'm going to have to do my best to use words to point to things that are *beyond* words. So I'll need to ask you to be a little patient and to allow some space for the information, ideas and perspectives within it to settle and find their proper place in their own time and way.

As I write this it feels like a rather unfashionable request. Who has time for that sort of thing these days? The thing is, though, I can't give you any simplistic answers—'Do this, do that and everything will be alright'—because there *aren't* any. And anyway, it's not that sort of book. It's a book about living, and life is a rich, complex and profound thing. That's the wonder of it. That's the point.

Let's begin, then, by taking some time to get a general sense of the territory we're going to explore, to plant some concepts and ideas and allow them to put down roots, grow and link up with each other.

Part One
Foundations

Chapter One
Discomfort and Ease

One day you wake up and say, 'I'm tired of mistreating myself.
—Marjorie Barstow[*]

I wonder what it's like to be you as you go about the day-to-day activities of your life. What qualities do you bring to the things you do and the people you interact with? The answer will change from activity to activity and moment to moment, but most of us have certain tendencies or habits that are particularly prominent—qualities and ways of being that we encounter in ourselves over and over again. So what does 'you' in action tend to look like? Do you tend to be rushed, lackadaisical, patient, intense, dogged or deliberate? Do you experience yourself physically as heavy, light, stiff, floppy, tight or collapsed? Do you meet the world and other people in ways that are forceful, reticent, domineering, retiring, responsive, rejecting, affirming or attuned?

Many of us become more set in our ways the older we get. Particular ways of being and acting become habitual. They become so comfortable and familiar that they come to seem inevitable, even if they cause a certain amount of discomfort or suffering to ourselves or those around us. They come to seem to be *us*, until we barely notice the state we're in and find it hard to imagine anything different.

I once had an Alexander Technique student who was in constant physical discomfort. His body was hunched

---

[*] Quoted by Bruce Fertman in *Teaching by Hand, Learning by Heart.*

and rigid, his muscles so shortened and stiff that even lying down on a table at the beginning of a lesson would cause him to cry out with pain. It was uncomfortable to be around. Every movement he made, and even the words he spoke, were forced and full of effort. He spent his days driving himself on, rushing from activity to activity—most of which weren't even necessary—never stopping, never letting his system come back to balance or allowing his body to reset, recover and find equilibrium.

This man could see, when it was pointed out to him, that this lifetime of heedless rushing and effort had a considerable bearing on his ongoing discomfort. And yet he struggled to stop doing it.

'It's who I am,' he said. 'It's what I do.'

He didn't want to change. Instead, he wanted me to tell him how he could carry on with his compulsive, driven state of being without experiencing the unpleasant side effects. It was more important to him to experience himself in a familiar way than it was to reduce the suffering resulting from the choices he made.

'How silly,' we might say.

And yet we all carry on like this in one way or another, at least some of the time. We all sometimes hold on to attitudes and ways of being which, deep down, we know cause us suffering and harm our relationships with others. All of us would sometimes like our problems to be taken away without having to fundamentally change anything in ourselves. Of course! Give us a daily exercise routine, or a meditation we can do once a day and then forget about, or a distraction, a holiday or even (whisper it quietly) a pill.

Just sometimes, though, something shifts. We reach a point where this is no longer good enough. We are through with it! We realise that we want things to be different in the future, and we want that enough that we're prepared to be different *ourselves*. We decide we are willing to be in the world in a new way.

Ease and Skill

In a way it's strange that a book about ease and skill should have to be written at all. Other animals seem to embody these qualities quite naturally and unselfconsciously much of the time without reading books about it. It's not difficult to see the startling contrast between most adult humans today and the delicate, lithe skilfulness and enjoyment of movement that other creatures spontaneously manifest for most of their lives. The grace, coordination and controlled power that a leopard exhibits when leaping across a river or that a group of dolphins display when corralling a school of mackerel are incredible to us. Each part of them seems to be integrated with every other part, their wishes and intentions, mind and body working effortlessly together as a whole. Everything flows.

Even people we think of as healthy and physically fit seldom attain the grace and ease that their pet cats and dogs exhibit as a matter of course. And yet, biologically, we're far more similar to other animals than we are different. We have similar sorts of cells, nerves, muscles and bones. If you cut us open, we look very much the same, and we originally evolved to deal with the same sorts of challenges presented by the natural world. And, in fact, that capacity for ease still seems to be latent within us. Many young children of about four or five move and carry themselves with a beautiful, upright, fluid alertness, evincing little of the tension, stiffness, slumping or collapse that most will manifest just a few years later. Some adults, too, never lose this quality—or at least can return to it in certain activities, such as the performing arts and sports. Think of the dancers Ginger Rogers and Fred Astaire, the pianist Arthur Rubinstein, the boxer Muhammad Ali or the tennis player Roger Federer. Often there's a subtle integration and fluidity to their movements. Even at rest there's a sense of ongoing alert aliveness—of their being poised and able to release easily into action in any direction at any moment. Something radically different seems to be happening for them—different not just from those of us who aren't elite performers but even from most of the other people in their field. Sometimes it looks as if they're playing a different game altogether.

I wonder if it would be fanciful to suggest that we're *supposed* to be that way—all of us, not just a talented few. It would be strange if, of all creatures, we were the only ones that evolved to move and hold themselves in a tense, rigid or collapsed way! People from cultures that have managed to retain some distance from modern ways of living and working sometimes seem to move with an easy, dynamic grace and skilfulness in contrast to the majority of contemporary humans. Perhaps many of our early human ancestors would also have tended to share a level of grace and ease in movement comparable to that displayed by the creatures of the natural world that they lived alongside.

Suppose you were to tentatively accept my suggestion that we originally evolved to exhibit a similar ease and grace to other members of the animal kingdom. In that case we must also be uniquely talented at messing things up for ourselves! How did things go so wrong for us? Later in this book I'll suggest that much of the problem originates from our all-too-human *cleverness*. Our capacity to think and reason, to learn new skills and to consciously shape our environment has made us uniquely powerful. But in the process, we've created technologies, cultures, social structures and ways of going about things which, though they bring certain benefits, put our minds, bodies and emotions under pressures they didn't originally evolve to deal with, causing physical and emotional discomfort and distress.

Beyond this, our ability to reason, think and learn enables us to intervene in the functioning of our bodies and minds far more than other animals can. We may respond to discomfort and distress we've created for ourselves by consciously or unconsciously attempting to make ourselves more comfortable through interfering in our body's workings without really understanding what we're doing. We may attempt to hold ourselves in certain attitudes or postures we believe to be beneficial, or forcefully direct our attention in the face of boredom and discomfort as we pursue our goals while using muscular tension to suppress unpleasant feelings and emotions. In the process, we unwittingly interfere with automatic systems in our bodies that are designed to manage essential functions such as postural stabilisation and support, movement, balance and breathing. Over time, this interference may become ingrained and habitual, undermining and compromising everything else that we do.

Fortunately, though, all is not lost! Once we understand the source of the trouble, we have a chance to put things right. In the later parts of this book we'll look at how we can learn to respond in wiser, more creative and skilful ways to the day-to-day challenges we face, and discover how we can learn to stop interfering and get out of the way so that our system can return to balance.

A Continuum of Discomfort and Ease

Pause for a moment and imagine a continuum. At one end are the easy, integrated, well-coordinated states that animals, young children and some skilled adults tend to exhibit, while at the other are more uncomfortable, tense, held or collapsed states that many of us experience a lot of the time.

When we're at the easy, well-coordinated end of the continuum, we tend to feel comfortable, light and free in ourselves. There's a sense of wholeness because our mind and body are working in harmony with each other. Our body tends to be experienced more as a source of delight than of stress or unpleasantness. Our movements are integrated, free and in harmony with our intentions, and everything we do tends to flow nicely with little energy wasted.

When we're at the other end of the continuum—in the more uncomfortable states characterised by stress and excess muscular contraction or by the muscular *under*-activation associated with slumping, heaviness and collapse—our movements are often unnecessarily tight and awkward. There's a lack of harmony between our body and our wishes and intentions. A great deal of energy is being wasted just hauling our weight around. Work and leisure activities tend to feel more difficult and less pleasant than they could, while excess muscular tension or collapse puts a lot of ongoing stress and strain on our body.

Many of us are so used to living like this that it comes to feel normal. It can be difficult to imagine anything different. We get so used to a lack of ease in ourselves that we barely notice it anymore, unless things get to the point—as they usually do in the end—where it begins to cause us some specific physical pain or difficulty. But, whether or not we're aware of it, all of us are at every moment occupying a place on this continuum between extreme discomfort and maximum ease.

Competence Versus Skill

Imagine two piano students, Bob and Sue. Both have been playing for a couple of years and have worked hard and learned some simple pieces. But when they sit down at the instrument they're very different to see and hear in action. Sue tends to inhabit the easy, integrated end of the continuum. She seems open and relaxed when she plays. There's a sense of flexibility and ease in her torso and arms and in the way she moves her hands and fingers. Her breathing is delicate and unlaboured, and her eyes move freely around the score enabling her to easily look ahead and back again to see what's coming up. Her whole body moves lightly and expressively to the music. The notes ripple along nicely and—though she's still something of a beginner—it sounds like she cares about and enjoys the music.

Bob, on the other hand, tends to inhabit the more uncomfortable end of the continuum. Though he's playing the right notes in the right order at the right time, there's a rather tight, worried quality about it all. His torso and arms are rigid, his eyes fixed and peering anxiously, unable to take in more than a note or two at a time. He holds his breath until the end of each phrase when he gasps another one in. Everything looks a bit heavy, effortful and anxious. It's a little unsettling to watch and listen to. The music doesn't flow freely; it's less musical and, in truth, he doesn't seem to be enjoying himself very much.

If we wanted to describe the difference between these two players, we might say that Bob's playing is more or less **competent**. He's playing the right notes, after all, and we can easily recognise the piece and hum along to it. Sue's playing, on the other hand, is **skilful**. She's not just getting the notes but doing so with a quality of ease, lightness and grace that infuses the music and her whole being as she plays.

How can we explain the discrepancy between these two? Perhaps, we might think, Bob doesn't have enough talent or isn't working hard enough. If only he'd been born with different genes or would practise the movements of his arms and fingers more often, repeating them over and over until they became ingrained, then he would, in the end, be able to make music in a more free and relaxed way like Sue. The trouble with this, though, is that Bob's difficulty has nothing to do with a lack of practice or talent. Playing the piano with a degree of skill is a challenge that most of us can get to grips with if we go about it in the right way. It doesn't take any unusual abilities. And Bob is keen to learn—he wants to play well and works just as hard as Sue. The key to the difference between the two of them lies at a deeper level, in the way that the underlying state of their system, and how they think about and use that system, supports or undermines what they're trying to achieve.

Any activity—whether it's as simple as standing up and walking across a room or as demanding as playing the piano—depends on much more fundamental abilities, such as how we focus our attention, how we deal with our body's responses to emotional stress, how we gain support and stability from our musculature, how we balance and how we coordinate our movements. If our attention is unfocused or over-focused, if we can't remain effortlessly upright and balanced in the field of gravity, skilfully coordinate our movements and regulate the stress and anxiety invoked by learning and performing, then we're going to struggle to reach our potential in complex activities that are built on these more basic abilities.

Endgaining

Often we tend to focus our attention on the most obvious parts of whatever activity we're engaged in, which is usually the concrete results we're hoping to achieve at the end of it, and we judge our performance entirely by those. We judge our piano-playing by whether it sounds right, with the correct notes in the correct order at the correct speed. We judge our tennis-playing by how hard and accurately we hit the ball and whether we can get it past our opponent. And of course these *are* essential aspects of these activities.

However, when we're *excessively* focused on these outward aspects of success we may fail to notice the wider impact of the mindset we're using as we attempt to achieve our aim. F.M. Alexander called this attitude **endgaining**. When we endgain, all we're thinking about is achieving the tangible goal—or 'end'—that we have in mind as quickly as possible. If I manage to balance on the bicycle and zoom along, or play a recognisable tune on the piano, or whack the ball across the net, I consider that a success. I have 'gained my end', and that is enough.

What is being missed, though, is *everything else that matters*. Am I taking care of myself as I do this thing, or am I storing up trouble for later? Does it feel good and expansive to be doing it this way? Am I being the sort of 'me' that I aspire to be, or am I being a rather uptight, driven and unhappy sort of me? Is the way I'm moving, balancing, breathing and focusing my awareness in the pursuit of my goal allowing my body to be as easy and free as it might be? Does it enable me to feel comfortable and secure? Does it allow for a sense of that flow, grace and ease characteristic of true skilfulness? Does it leave me able to access my authentic feelings and emotions and bring them to whatever I'm doing?

How much nicer it would be if we could achieve our aims while taking care of ourselves as best as we are able! How wonderful if the results we gained came about precisely *because* we were open, balanced, happy, curious and free in ourselves as we progressed towards them. How lovely if, by taking care to allow our body to function with delicacy, subtlety and refinement, we found a completely new and unexpected depth of skill in which that subtlety and refinement were deliciously expressed in what we were doing!

One of the fundamental aims of this book is to help you become aware of the way you go about things and of how this affects you. My hope is that this will begin to open up a space where you can start to make different choices—ones that are more in accord with well-being, with your deeper goals, and with the way your body and mind evolved to be.

Chapter Two
Three Views of the Self

Do I contradict myself?
Very well then I contradict myself,
(I am large, I contain multitudes.)
—WALT WHITMAN, 'Song of Myself'

There's a contradiction, a question and perhaps a little joke or two lurking in the title of this book. *A User's Guide to the Self*. Who is this 'self' we're talking about—and who is the 'user' who is using it?

'Self' is a word we tend to use without thinking too much about it. It's easy to take for granted that we know what it means and who 'ourself' is. But as soon as we dig a little deeper, we come across questions and contradictions that can take us to the edges of science and philosophy. F.M. Alexander, for example, defined the self as the totality of the person—the mind and body considered together as an indivisible whole. That makes a certain kind of sense. If I'm thinking about 'you', I will probably have a single image in mind which includes your body, your personality and your thoughts and feelings as I experience them. I wouldn't think of you and your body separately. I'd think of them as aspects of one being—yourself. And, in fact, we can see that our thoughts, feelings and body *are* deeply and inextricably connected. You only have to wish to raise your hand or nod your head and it happens. Every emotion you feel affects, and is in turn affected by, numerous other functions throughout your body. When you're happy, your torso spontaneously becomes more upright and open, your eyes sparkle and your face relaxes and becomes more friendly and approachable. Maybe your heart rate settles a little and your breathing becomes freer and easier too. When you're sad, on the other hand, your shoulders tend to sag and collapse; your face becomes heavy as your eyes falter and fall. Conversely, your thoughts and how you see yourself and the world around you are deeply conditioned by how you experience your body from moment to moment. It's hard to think light, free, optimistic thoughts if your body is slumped, collapsed or heavy.

So we can think of ourself as one unified mind–body, a single integrated organism. I tend to refer to this integrated being as the 'whole self', or simply the Self, with a capital letter.

It's extraordinary to think what this organism is capable of! It can stand up, walk about and sense its surroundings in minute detail. It can reach out with its hands and manipulate objects in infinite ways. It can not only imagine new things but bring them into being. It can tell jokes, laugh, sing and make love. It's capable of wonderful athletic and artistic feats that embody both great strength and tremendous sensitivity.

Most of the time we don't give much thought to how much has to happen under the surface to enable us to do even the simplest everyday things like sitting, walking and communicating with each other, let alone the more demanding ones. Nevertheless, everything we do requires a complex interaction of perception, thought, emotion, muscle and bone. Given how intricate our mind–body system is—and how precariously we're balanced on two legs much of the time—it's a miracle that we can do anything useful at all. The fact that we *can* raises some intriguing questions about control. How is all the complex muscular and sensory activity that is required to move and coordinate ourselves in the Earth's gravitational field guided and directed? If the Self includes everything that we are, who or what is controlling it?

In reality, even though seen from one perspective our mind and body are a single unified being, we frequently experience ourselves rather differently from this. Often there seems to be an observer—an 'I' or 'me'—who can look at 'its' body objectively and even (somewhat paradoxically) at its own thoughts and feelings. I can admire my body or complain about it as if it were a somewhat tiresome family member rather than something I *am*. I may decide that it's too thin or fat, or tired, or old, and I may even say to myself that I'll try to correct and improve these shortcomings. I can ask my body to move, jump up and down or sing, and it obeys. I can think about my arm or my leg and decide to move them about like a puppeteer pulling the strings.

In this book I'll refer to these deliberate actions of the I as **voluntary** activity, which is undertaken by the **voluntary self** or, more colloquially, simply as *your* decisions and actions which are performed by *you*.

Some might claim there's an illusory quality to this sense of being a separate me—that it's a chimaera created by the mind. Many spiritual traditions have suggested this, and contemporary brain science tends to do so too. But if it *is* an illusion it's a very convincing, powerful and necessary one. Without a sense of 'me' and what I'm up to I can't make plans, consider the past or future, or work out how to achieve a goal. The sense of being a separate, thinking, reasoning self is essential for me to take intelligent, deliberate action.[*]

Although this kind of voluntary action is essential, it's insufficient on its own to control all the intricacies of muscles and movement needed for us to live and act effectively in the world. Imagine if, in order to stand up, you had to voluntarily control every single muscle that was involved. Even if you could do it you would have little mental capacity left for anything else. Fortunately, though, you *don't* have to, because underlying and enabling our voluntary actions are all sorts of helpful things going on that arise automatically, independently of our conscious will.

We all know that things are going on in our bodies that we never learned and don't deliberately do. Our heart beats whether we ask it to or not, our lungs breathe, our eyes automatically blink away tears and dust, and our throat swallows to clear phlegm and keep our airway open. Other responses assist with stability, balance, emotional regulation, perception and movement. These movements, processes and reactions arise from our mind–body system as a whole through the interaction of nerves, reflexes, muscles, sense organs and activity in both high- and low-level parts of the brain. In this book I'll refer to these kinds of automatic, self-regulating responses as the **spontaneous** activity of your 'system' or, more colloquially, of your 'body' because a lot of the time that's exactly how we experience it—our body is doing something on its own, independently of our conscious intentions and will.

Without the constant help of these spontaneous regulating and controlling actions of the body we would die

---

[*] F.M. Alexander talked in terms of 'using' ourselves, pointing out that we can do so skilfully—leading to ease and effectiveness in our activities—or less skilfully, causing tension, discomfort and stress.

in an instant, and we'd be unable to take even the simplest deliberate action.

Some of the most important things that these spontaneous functions help to regulate and control are:

- Breathing, blood flow and digestion

- The basic emotional responses that evolved to help us survive in the face of threats and opportunities in our environment

- Our ability to sense ourselves and the world about us, and to orient ourselves to our surroundings

- The muscular tone needed to stabilise our joints

- Our system's ability to mobilise that stabilisation to support us so that we can remain upright in the field of gravity

- The continual subtle adjustments needed to keep us balanced so we don't fall over

- The coordinations needed to enable complex, multi-joint movements

It's helpful to know about these spontaneous functions, because the way we relate to them has a great influence on the degree of freedom and ease our system is able to manifest from moment to moment. In the next few chapters we'll learn more about how they work, and about how their activity can either support or undermine us in our journey towards skilfulness and ease.

Chapter Three
Blood Flow and Breathing

Breathing, blood circulation and digestion are our basic life support systems, working together to ensure that our blood is absorbing oxygen and nutrients, that these are taken where they're needed, and that waste products such as lactic acid and carbon dioxide are expelled from the body. Together they're controlled by a network of nerves and lower brain centres called the **autonomic nervous system**.

At the centre of this system is the heart, which—despite being only the size of our fist—pumps about five litres of blood around our body every minute even when we're resting. It sends blood through the pulmonary artery to our lungs where oxygen is absorbed and carbon dioxide is expelled. The freshly oxygenated blood is returned to the heart via the pulmonary vein from where it's sent, via a network of arteries and tiny capillaries, to our muscles and internal organs.

Our arteries can contract to regulate blood pressure throughout our body, while pressure in the capillaries is regulated by little bands of muscles called precapillary sphincters, so that every muscle and organ gets just the amount of blood it needs.

On its way round the body, the blood passes through our digestive system. Here it absorbs nutrients from the small intestine while the liver and kidneys filter out waste. These processes require a lot of blood—generally about twenty to twenty-five per cent of the heart's output, increasing substantially after a meal. The used blood returns to the heart through our veins before being taken once more to the lungs as the cycle begins again.

Our breathing, cardiovascular and digestive functions work together, constantly adjusting to ensure the body has the energy it needs to deal with whatever situations we're facing. These adjustments are controlled by the autonomic nervous system which is divided into two branches: the **sympathetic** and the **parasympathetic**. The sympathetic branch is responsible for increasing our levels of energy and arousal when needed, while the parasympathetic branch is responsible for calming us down.

The more active we are the more oxygenated blood our muscles need, so the faster and harder our heart needs to pump and the faster we need to breathe. These changes are facilitated by the sympathetic nervous system which alters our breathing pattern, increases our heart rate, causes our arteries and veins to contract to increase our blood pressure, and diverts blood from the digestive system to our muscles and lungs where it's most needed. When we're ready to return to rest, our parasympathetic nervous system activates to reverse this process—calming our breathing, dilating our arteries and veins to lower our blood pressure, lowering our heart rate and directing blood back to the intestines and digestive system.

Because of its role in regulating our energy and arousal levels, the autonomic nervous system also plays an essential role in our emotional responses. When we're afraid, for example, our limbic brain, where our emotions are processed, activates the sympathetic branch to arouse energy to prepare us for fight or flight. When the danger passes it activates the parasympathetic branch to calm us down again. We'll learn more about our basic emotional responses and how they effect our minds and bodies in the next chapter.

More About the Breath

We can't directly control our heartbeat, blood circulation or digestive system—they go on automatically. But although much of the time the breath goes on automatically too, we can also deliberately control it. We can choose to interrupt it for a while—to speed it up, slow it down or make it deeper or shallower. We can prioritise different parts of our breathing mechanism, breathing low down from the diaphragm or higher up with the ribs. We can choose to breathe through our nose, our mouth or both alternately.

This ability to control our breath voluntarily is essential for activities like swimming, diving, talking, singing and eating, and it can also help us coordinate our movements in rhythmic activities like running. We'll see later that our ability to control our breath can also help us to voluntarily regulate our level of emotional arousal due to the breath's connection to our emotional states via the autonomic nervous system. Generally, though, it's best to allow the breath to self-regulate. The body knows much better than we do how to breathe! Can you imagine a cat or a dog trying to breathe 'correctly'? Most of the time it's just as absurd for us to do so.

High- and Low-Arousal Breathing

Many structures in the body support and enable breathing. Some of the most important ones are the lungs (which take up most of the space within the ribcage), the ribs, the intercostal muscles which run diagonally between each rib helping them to rise and fall, and the diaphragm which is a dome-shaped muscle spanning the bottom of the chest cavity, separating it from the abdomen (fig. 1).

For air to be drawn into the lungs, the space inside the chest cavity needs to increase. This can happen in two main ways. The diaphragm can contract, flattening out and descending to create space above it, or the ribs can rise to create space by expanding the ribcage.

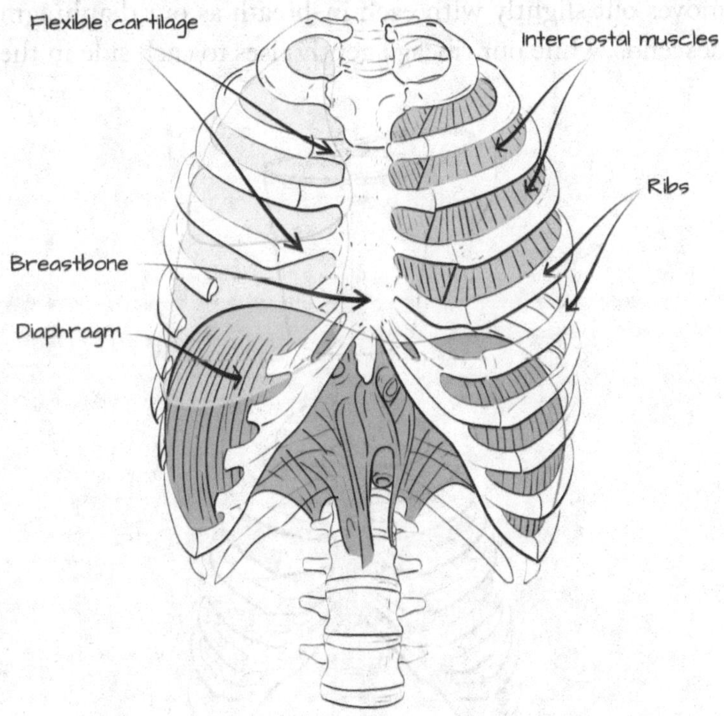

Fig. 1. The Breathing Mechanism

Like all bodily functions, breathing is adaptive, spontaneously becoming faster, slower, deeper or shallower depending on how much oxygen we need from moment to moment. To help with this, different breathing patterns spontaneously activate depending on the situation.

Suppose our system is in a calm, relaxed state and we feel safe and secure. In that case our breathing tends to adopt its 'low-arousal' mode, involving gentle, blended movements of the diaphragm, belly and ribs. These movements are focused quite low down in our torso. Our belly moves out slightly with each in-breath as our diaphragm descends, while our ribcage gently rises to each side in the

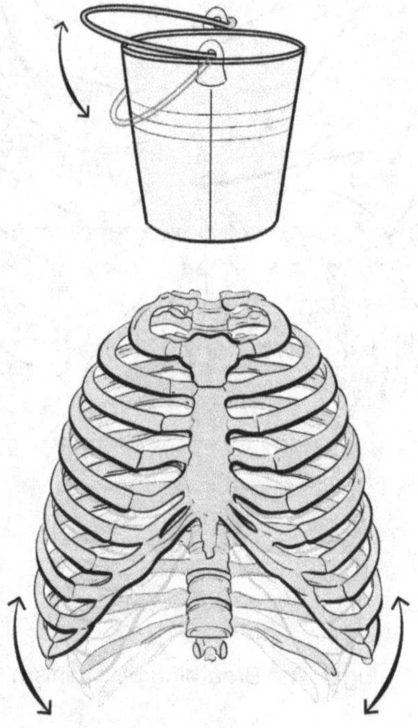

Fig. 2. The Bucket Handle Movement (front view)

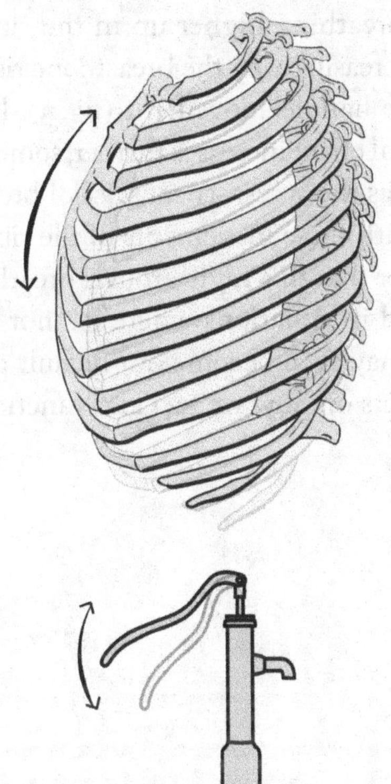

Fig. 3. The Pump Handle Movement (side view)

'bucket handle' movement (fig. 2). If we become more active these movements may become bigger, but so long as we remain calm and relaxed they retain the same quiet, blended quality.

If, on the other hand, we become aroused by fear, anxiety or heavy physical exertion, our breathing pattern spontaneously changes, becoming shallower and faster to recycle the air in our lungs as quickly as possible. The abdominal muscles contract and brace around the abdominal organs preventing the diaphragm from descending, pushing the movements of breathing higher up in the ribcage where they're driven increasingly by the breastbone rising and falling in the 'pump handle' movement (fig. 3). If emotional arousal or physical effort increases further, some of our neck muscles (known as the accessory muscles of breathing) may join in to help with these movements of the ribcage.

We'll see later that this high-arousal breathing pattern can get triggered in situations where it's not appropriate or helpful, and may even become our default pattern with detrimental effects on how we feel and function.

Chapter Four

Primitive Emotional Responses

Humans have complex emotional lives compared to other animals, but our emotions are still built on primitive survival responses we share with them, such as fear, anger, excitement, disgust, sexual arousal, curiosity and contentment. These can get triggered automatically well before we've had time to consciously think about what's happening. This makes sense. Many of the situations our ancestors faced in the natural world demanded immediate action. When danger or opportunity arose there was often no time to think before responding. There needed to be an instant arousal of energy for pursuit, fighting or escape.

We can categorise our emotional responses in terms of whether they are high or low arousal and whether we experience them as pleasant or unpleasant. Anger, fear and excitement are generally high arousal. They wake us up and make us ready for action. Contentment and sadness are more towards the low-arousal end of the scale, while sexual arousal can be high, low, or a combination of the two. Fear and sadness feel unpleasant, excitement, contentment and sexual arousal feel pleasant, and anger can feel pleasant or unpleasant depending on the circumstances.

Fear: Fight, Flight, Freeze and Flop

The primary aim of all creatures is to not get eaten, and various spontaneous emotional reactions evolved to help protect us from this fate. Imagine being an early human walking through the forest. Suddenly you glimpse a movement behind some bushes. Good grief!—a leopard. Your limbic brain releases a flood of adrenaline and noradrenaline into your bloodstream, stimulating your sympathetic nervous system to burst into action, raising your heart rate, shifting your breathing to its high-arousal pattern to rapidly oxygenate your blood, and diverting blood from your digestive system to your muscles giving rise to a lurching feeling of butterflies in the stomach. Your musculature spontaneously tightens to provide rigidity, stability and power for self-defence or flight. Your senses become heightened and focused on the threat while blood flow decreases to the parts of your brain concerned with thought and reflection, and increases to those that help you take instinctive action.

If your brain decides you may be able to successfully flee the situation, an intense feeling of fear will be aroused to motivate you to run away. If it seems that a better option may be to confront the danger head-on, you feel a burst of anger encouraging you to fight furiously for survival. These spontaneous reactions make up the **fight–flight** response.

But what if the leopard hasn't seen you yet? Perhaps neither fight nor flight is the best solution in the circumstances. Either would draw attention to you, so your limbic brain triggers a **freeze** response instead. You're still quivering with energy, and if an opportunity to escape arose, all that energy would be released in a frantic, chaotic rush for safety. But for now you are immobilised, stuck to the spot, literally unable to move or even speak.

Perhaps, though, the leopard senses your presence anyway. It stops, looks straight at you, and utters a low growl. Too late to run, hopeless to fight! It comes padding towards you, step by step. As a final resort, your brain triggers a **flop** response. You fall to the ground and go limp as your brain functions start to shut down. This may still help you because many wild animals won't attack a creature that already appears to be dead. Either the predator will lose interest and move on, or this final throw of the dice will fail—in which case, at least the shutdown of your mental capacities will help to reduce your awareness of the situation.[*]

These primitive defensive responses originally evolved to protect us in life-or-death situations, but they are also the basis of our instinctive reaction to *any* kind of threat. They get triggered in less intense ways whenever we're anxious or afraid, even if the danger isn't life-threatening or happening in the here and now. They can be triggered, for example, in response to worries about what might happen in the future, or in response to threats to our social status, possessions, health or relationships. It's helpful to understand these responses and their effects because when they get activated they have a significant impact on how our brains and bodies function. We'll be learning a lot more about this as we go on.

---

[*] People who have experienced very traumatic events such as violence or sexual assault often report these freeze and flop responses. In such situations they may be quite literally unable to move and there's nothing that can be done about it—their nervous system has made the choice for them. This inability to respond at the time can give rise to feelings of deep shame afterwards as the person blames themself for not fighting back or removing themselves from danger.

Excitement

Excitement is a high-energy state that has both similarities to, and differences from, the fight–flight response. Its origins may lie in the hunting instinct, where it arouses energy and enthusiasm for the chase. Nowadays we can have similar exhilarating experiences as we marshal our skills in sporting activities or artistic performance.

When we become excited, our limbic brain activates our sympathetic nervous system, raising our heart rate and breathing and diverting blood from our digestive system to our muscles just as it does with the fight–flight response. But excitement differs from that response in important ways. Because it's not a response to a threat it doesn't arouse protective muscular bracing or spontaneous narrowing of our field of attention. Generally when we're excited, our visual field remains open, wide and free so that we can keep track of the big picture, strategise and see what the rest of our 'pack' is doing around us. We may feel pleasant and stirring emotions, such as glee, camaraderie or joyful anticipation. At the same time, though, the parts of our brain concerned with deliberate thought and reason may become less active as our system focuses on taking action in the moment, giving rise to the possibility of being carried away by our excitement and getting into situations we later regret!

Engagement, Interest and Curiosity

Occupying the middle ground between high- and low-arousal states are those, such as interest and curiosity, in which we're active and engaged in what we're doing but without any great sense of urgency. In these states our nervous system is in balance. We're gently, pleasantly alert, our field of awareness is wide and receptive, and we have full access to our higher mental faculties so we can easily bring thought and consideration to whatever we're up to. Such states are ideal for learning, social interaction and most day-to-day activities. If we're occupied with a work project, in conversation with a friend or practising skills like music or art, it helps to be in an alert, present state of mind with sufficient energy to focus on what we're doing but without excessive muscular tension or emotional intensity.

Low-Arousal States

Animals have a natural rhythm of arousal and relaxation which they follow throughout the day. There will be times they are active—hunting, seeking food, exploring, mating and raising young—and times when they're resting and recuperating. Many of us humans have become adept at ignoring or overriding our body when it signals that it's time to stop and rest. But most animals switch naturally and easily between high- and low-arousal states. After eating or exerting themselves they will tend to stop and rest quietly.

In these calm states, the parasympathetic nervous system is dominant, quietening and regulating the breath and heart rate and diverting blood from the muscles to the digestive system. This state is called **rest-and-digest** and is accompanied by pleasant feelings of comfort and relaxation. It's the feeling you might get on a warm summer evening after a good meal with friends—time to stretch out and lounge for a bit with no particular agenda as your body recharges.

There are also low-arousal states, however, that are less

pleasant to experience. If we are sick or injured, or have suffered an emotional wound, for example, our system may generate unpleasant feelings, such as fatigue, vulnerability or sadness that force us to stop, withdraw and find space for integration and healing.

Chapter Five
Sensing and Attention

To live and function in the world we need to be aware of ourselves and our surroundings, and this begins with our senses. The most familiar of these are touch, taste, sight, sound and smell. They're called the **exteroceptive** senses because they mostly give us information about things that are external to us. But there are also many other, lesser-known ones. There is our **vestibular** sense, for example, which uses tiny organs in our inner ear to give us information about how we are moving through space. Then there are the various **interoceptive** senses which tell us what's happening inside us such as our body temperature, feelings of hunger and thirst, movements in our digestion system and our state of emotional arousal. And finally there are the **proprioceptive** senses which enable us to sense the position of our joints, to feel how much muscular effort we're applying from moment to moment, and to sense our movements (kinaesthesia).

Scientists make a distinction between sensing and perceiving. For them, sensing refers to the brain's reception of raw sensory data whereas perception is how it puts that data together into a coherent picture of ourselves and the world around us. But we don't usually experience things like this in everyday life. Sensing and perception seem to be all-of-a-piece. Right now, for example, I'm aware that I'm sitting at my desk. There's a vivid sensation of having a body, of the room around me, of the open window and of traffic passing in the rain. If my partner comes in and touches my arm, the contact is experienced vividly *there*, on my skin, rather than as a process happening inside my head. So in this book I'll use the word 'sensing' in a more colloquial, everyday way to refer to the whole experience of being aware of our body and the world through the senses.

The Visual System

Smell is the primary sense for many animals, and their relationship with the world is organised around it. Think about a dog or a pig. Much of the time they literally follow their noses. For humans, though, the primary sense is vision. The priority of our visual sense is so deeply hard-wired that even people who were born blind will spontaneously move their heads towards objects of interest as if they were looking at them, and when there's a conflict between what our eyes and another of the senses is telling us, the brain will generally assume the eyes are correct.

Though we experience looking at the things around us as a simple act, it's actually an extremely complex phenomenon. Whenever we shift our gaze we trigger an extraordinary dance of spontaneous movement, coordination and balance which happens without conscious thought or effort. Think about turning to look at something behind you. Numerous changes throughout your body need to be precisely coordinated to enable you to do this. Your head needs to turn towards the object you are interested in while keeping your eyes level with the horizon. Your eyes must converge on the object and then focus on it using the tiny, delicate ciliary muscles around each lens. Other tiny muscles expand or contract the iris allowing just the right amount of light onto the retina. In the meantime, turning your head will have affected your centre of gravity requiring shifts in muscle tone throughout your body to keep you stabilised and balanced, while continuous compensations will need to be made to keep your eyes on their target despite any ongoing movements of the object or yourself. Think about how, if we make a dash for a train, our gaze can remain fixed on the door we're aiming for without deliberate effort.

We couldn't possibly manage all this voluntarily—it's only possible because we have spontaneous systems to help. We have reflexes, for example, that maintain our head in a level position despite movements of our body. Other reflexes keep our eyes fixed on the object of interest by moving them in the opposite direction when we turn our head. Still others focus our lenses, adjust the size of our pupils to adapt to brightness or darkness, and cause tiny shifts of our eyeballs to stabilise the image. Further systems help to keep our body as a whole stabilised and balanced while all this is going on. We'll learn more about these in the next few chapters.

Orienting

As well as playing an essential role in organising our ability to look at things and stabilise our gaze, our system can also make spontaneous decisions about what we should be looking *at*. For example, whenever our brain senses a threatening sound or movement, or something unfamiliar and unexpected, our head and eyes automatically turn to look at it long before we've had a chance to consciously evaluate what's happening. This is called the **involuntary orienting response.**

In addition to this, our visual system is designed to respond to our *conscious* interest. When we're interested in something, we don't need to think about moving our head and eyes to look at it. Our interest and curiosity make our head and eyes turn towards it without us having to deliberately guide them there. This tendency for our system to spontaneously turn our gaze towards the things we are interested in is called the **voluntary orienting response**.

Concentration and the Field of Attention

As well as orienting ourselves towards the things we need to look at, we also need to be able to focus our vision and other senses to include and exclude things from our awareness. To understand more about how this works, let's imagine again that you're an early human walking through the forest.

The birds are calling from the trees as you head to the river to fish. There doesn't seem to be anything dangerous about so your field of attention is wide, open and free, your vision and hearing moving lightly from thing to thing, receptive to the whole gamut of sights and sounds around you as you notice and enjoy the physical sensations of moving and being in a body. The rich information your system is receiving from all these sensory channels enables your spontaneous systems for postural support, balance and movement to work at their best, helping your movements to be graceful, easy and free.

This ease and freedom is particularly helped by the wide, open state of your field of vision. Your visual field is organised into two zones. There is a very small **central zone**, which is the part that is most sensitive to visual detail, and there is a much larger **peripheral zone** surrounding it which is more sensitive to movement while still giving you a rough impression of shape and colour. The peripheral zone has particularly strong neural connections to parts of the brain that help you balance, orient yourself and move through space. Having a broad field of vision gives your system more of this important information.

Let's now say you come to the river and settle down to fish. Your field of attention becomes rather more focused than it was when you were walking. You pay more attention to the task and less to the forest around you. But your vision and other senses are still relatively open and free, moving lightly back and forth from the rod in your hands to the river, the line, the fish, yourself, your surroundings and your footing on the bank.

The ability to focus on a task while still keeping a relatively open, flexible field of attention is an essential part of skilful activity. Whether we're sitting or standing quietly, walking alone or engaged in more demanding tasks, our attention needs to be receptive and free, giving us the detailed sensory information we need to do the task, as well as the overall awareness of ourselves and our surroundings which helps our system to organise in an easy, integrated way.

Unfortunately, many of us have lost the knack of establishing and maintaining a state of free, open attention, tending to habitually adopt rather intent, narrowly focused and fixed states of awareness instead. Let's go back to the forest to begin to get an idea of where these over-intent, narrowed-down states originate from.

Voluntary Versus Spontaneous Concentration
Imagine you've finished fishing and are walking home in the gathering dusk when, out of the corner of your eye,

your system senses a flash of movement between some trees. Your head snaps spontaneously towards it and your field of attention narrows to a point, concentrating all your awareness on that one potentially vital spot—eyes and ears straining to sense what's there. For the moment your peripheral vision and awareness of your body is lost, but it doesn't matter because right now survival is more important than ease and gracefulness. Without thinking, you stop dead in your tracks as muscles spontaneously brace throughout your body—particularly in your eyes, head and neck—and your breath tightens, becoming shallower and perhaps even momentarily stopping altogether. These changes help to stabilise your visual system, reducing unnecessary body movements to help you see any danger more clearly. As a bonus, your stillness makes you less conspicuous to a potential predator.

But it seems you're in luck. After a moment you realise there's nothing there. It was just a chance pattern of light and shade. You breathe out with a sigh of relief, shake yourself briefly and laugh, your head, neck and eyes unfreezing and letting go back into a state of free and open attention as you head lightly for home.

Interestingly, the mechanisms that underlie this spontaneous concentration which arises in response to a threat also seem to underlie our ability to concentrate *voluntarily*, such as when we *choose* to focus intently and exclusively on an object or task. Whenever we concentrate voluntarily on something, there's an accompanying stiffening and fixing of our visual system and breathing. Our eyes, head, neck and breath tighten just as they do when we're in physical danger. Crucially, this happens *even if we're concentrating with a sense other than vision*—for example if we're straining to hear a faint sound in the distance, or if we're turning our attention inwards to focus intently on a bodily sensation or on our mental world of thoughts and images as we might if we were trying to solve a difficult maths problem in our heads.

While voluntary concentration is occasionally useful (such as when we need to work with tiny objects, or if we need to pick out a small detail from many competing stimuli), many of us have got into the habit of concentrating far more than we need to, in situations where it's *not* necessary or helpful. The muscular tension and rigidity that is evoked by this, together with the accompanying loss of peripheral vision, deeply compromise our ability to move and do things with ease and skilfulness.

Fortunately, though, as we'll see later, this involuntary muscular fixing and holding can also help us to let go of our habits of unnecessary concentration because, once we get used to spotting it, it can act as a clear, easy-to-notice indicator that we're focussing our attention more intently than we should be. We'll find out more about how these unnecessary habits of concentration develop, and how we can learn to let go of them, later on in the book.

Chapter Six
Stabilisation

Our bodies are *agile*, enabling us to adopt an infinite variety of shapes and movements. We can use our arms to grasp and manipulate objects, to support our weight, and to pull or push ourselves towards or away from things. We can use them to gesture and gesticulate and to wrap around those we love. We can use our feet and legs to clamber, climb and kick as well as to get around the world through walking, running, swimming and other methods of loco-motion. We can use our heads to look around us, to balance things on and to push things with. We can even use our mouths to hold things, leaving our hands free for other tasks. Our torsos can wriggle, bend and stretch in all directions, while allowing us to breathe and supporting the weight of our limbs and head.

This tremendous agility is made possible by the articulated structure of our skeleton. Its rigid bones give us our form while the many joints between them allow for movement. But before we even begin to do anything useful, those moveable joints need to be **stabilised** by our muscles so they don't collapse under our own weight. This stabilisation of individual joints needs to be coordinated throughout the body so that our structure as a whole is **supported** in the face of gravity. And having found this stabilisation and support, we need to be able to maintain our **balance** so we don't fall over.

I will be using these words—stabilisation, support and balance—in those very specific ways throughout this book. Stabilisation refers to the *way in which* our muscles activate to maintain the individual joints of our skeleton in whatever position is needed from moment to moment. Support refers to how this stabilisation is *organised throughout the body* to keep us upright in the face of gravity and any other forces that impinge on us. And balance is the way we remain aligned in the field of gravity so that this stabilised, supported structure doesn't topple and fall.

Two Types of Stabilisation

Stabilisation is a fundamental bodily function, and the way it is achieved significantly affects how easy and comfortable we feel in ourselves, and the degree of skilfulness we can bring to our activities. Generally speaking, our muscles can stabilise our joints in one of two ways. They can work **dynamically**, adjusting sensitively to provide the precise amount of muscle tone needed from moment to moment, or they can **brace**, tightening against each other to hold our joints rigidly in position.

Muscles can only apply force in one direction. They can pull inwards but they can't push outwards. Because of this they're always arranged in opposing pairs or groups. Your elbow joint is a simple example. The biceps contract to bend your elbow, and the triceps contract to straighten it again. A more complex example can be seen in the muscles that bend your torso forwards and backwards. In this case, several muscles in your back contract simultaneously to bend your spine backwards, and several others down the front of your body contract to bend it forwards.

Try bending and tensing your elbow to show off your

biceps muscle like children do. This braces and locks your elbow joint, making it rigid. Your biceps and triceps muscles are contracting simultaneously, over-tightening and clamping down against each other. It's a bit like a tent pole supported by guy ropes. The more you tighten the ropes, the more firmly and rigidly the pole will be held until you can push it quite hard in any direction and be unable to move it.

In a similar way, when our muscles brace our joints, those joints become very stiff, enabling them to maintain their position in the face of a wide range of forces without any need for moment-to-moment adjustment. If you were to brace your elbow and ask a friend to take your hand and try to bend or straighten your arm, they'd be able to pull and push with varying degrees of force—from very lightly to quite firmly—and your elbow would remain in position without you needing to change the amount of effort you were applying to keep it there.

Now let's think about something different. Imagine playing a simple game with a friend. You stand opposite each other, your arms raised, making palm-to-palm contact, both of you leaning forwards slightly so that you have to push a little with your arms to prevent you from falling forwards into each other.

The idea of the game is that your friend slowly moves their hands about while you try to keep yours in contact with them, tracking their movements as closely and delicately as you can. Because you're leaning into each other, the temptation might be to brace your arm muscles for security, but this won't help you to play the game well because it would cause you to freeze and tighten up. To follow them sensitively and accurately—neither lagging behind nor getting ahead—you would need to *exactly match* the forces being met, continuously adjusting from moment to moment, using just the right amount of force so that you neither fall into them nor push yourself awkwardly away, seamlessly switching from muscle to muscle as needed to delicately track their movements. Now, rather than bracing, your muscles are working *dynamically*.

Spontaneous Stabilisation Strategies

We have roughly 650 skeletal muscles moving about 350 joints that are in constantly changing relationship to each other and to gravity. Think how overwhelming it would be if we had to consciously and deliberately manage the continuous shifts of muscle tone needed to stabilise this structure. Fortunately, though, we don't have to, because most of it is taken care of automatically. If you reach out your hand to pick something up, for example, you don't need to think about simultaneously tightening various muscles in your back and legs so they can support the sudden weight of your now-extended arm. Your body does it for you. Whenever we're upright, numerous muscles are spontaneously adjusting from moment to moment to keep us stabilised and supported in the field of gravity.

In the examples above, you voluntarily braced your elbow, and voluntarily used dynamic stabilisation as you moved your hands and arms about to follow your friend's movements. But your body also *spontaneously* adopts these two contrasting modes as it stabilises and supports you, choosing one or the other according to the needs and demands of the moment.

When our system organises stabilisation in a responsive, dynamic way we are left open, sensitive, easy and free—the same qualities we may notice in a beautifully coordinated cat or a skilled and refined sportsperson or musician. This is comfortable and efficient because energy isn't being wasted by muscles tightening against each other, while the sensitivity, responsiveness and economy that accompany dynamic stabilisation help us perform better at skilled activities like music, dance and sports. Given its many advantages and its prevalence in animals, young children and skilful adults, it's likely that we evolved for dynamic stabilisation to be our system's default mode: it's the way things are supposed to work most of the time.

Despite the advantages of dynamic stabilisation, though, there are still times when it's appropriate and necessary for our system to spontaneously stabilise our joints by bracing instead. We've met some of these already:

- Our muscles spontaneously brace when we're fearful or **anxious** to prepare us for fight or flight or to make us freeze.

- Bracing is evoked whenever we **concentrate**.

- Bracing often happens naturally in activities that require tiny movements and extreme **steadiness**, such as threading a needle.

- Our muscles brace for stability if our system senses we're unbalanced and in danger of **falling**.

- Finally, our muscles spontaneously brace for stability when they're put under significant **load**, such as when we lift or push heavy weights, protecting us from collapse or damage if the load shifts unexpectedly.

One of the key themes in this book is that although these spontaneous bracing responses are basically healthy and helpful, many of us get into habits and ways of being that constantly inadvertently trigger them when they're *not* helpful, causing unnecessary tension in almost everything we do. We'll discover more about how this happens as we go on through the book.

Chapter Seven
Support

Stabilisation is an essential bodily function, but it's not much use unless it's coordinated throughout the body to keep us upright in the field of gravity.

Many of us have got into the habit of supporting our structure by bracing our muscles, but it's better if we can allow our system to support us sensitively and dynamically, letting it spontaneously adjust our musculature as needed from moment to moment. It's extraordinary that our body can to this in spite of our numerous joints and the precarious, unstable nature of our two-legged, upright stance. To understand what makes it possible, we'll need to begin by looking at a bit of anatomy, and particularly at the structure of our skeleton (this information will also be useful in other ways as we go on through the book).

The Parts of the Skeleton

We can divide our bones into two main groups: the **axial** skeleton and the **appendicular** skeleton. The axial skeleton consists of the bones that occupy the centre line of the body—the skull, spine and ribcage. The appendicular skeleton consists of the limbs, and the pelvis and shoulder girdle which connect them to the axial skeleton (fig. 4).

The Axial Skeleton

The **spine** is the most important part of the axial skeleton and the most fundamental structural element of the body.

It comprises thirty-three bones that together form a single flexible column (fig. 5). It can twist and bend in all directions while also being strong enough to support the weight of our arms, torso, head and ribcage, and the movements of breathing. It settles naturally into a gentle double curve, which helps it absorb jolts and shocks.

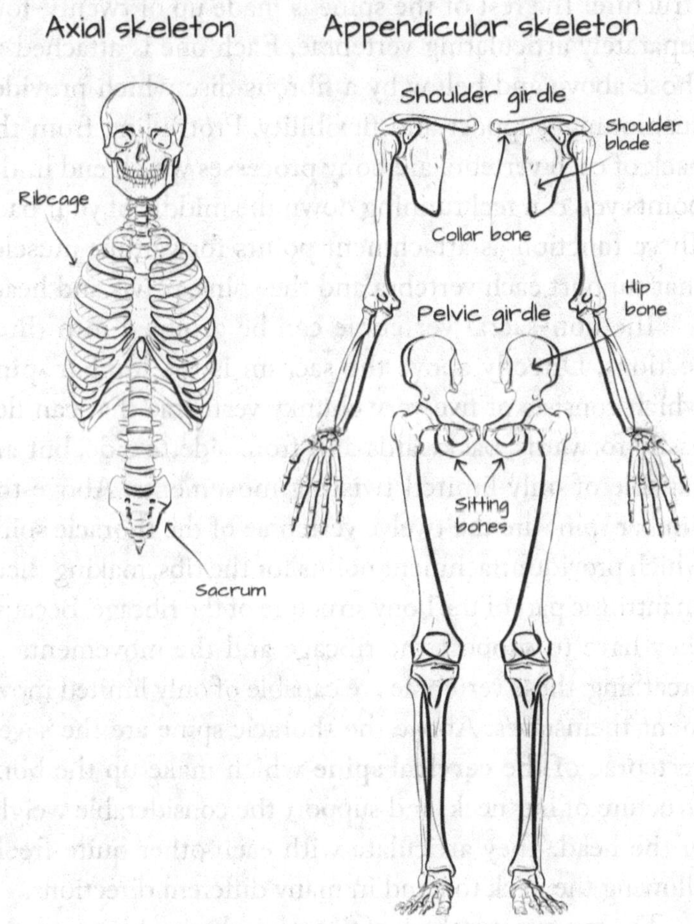

Fig. 4. Axial and Appendicular Skeletons

The **coccyx** is the lowest part of the spine. It's a tiny vestigial tail left over from our evolutionary ancestors. Above the coccyx is the **sacrum**, which consists of five vertebrae fused together to create a single triangular-shaped bone which is so securely attached to the pelvis that it makes sense to think of them as a single, integrated structure. The rest of the spine is made up of twenty-four separately articulating vertebrae. Each one is attached to those above and below by a fibrous disc which provides cushioning, support and flexibility. Protruding from the back of each vertebra are bony **processes** which end in the points you can feel running down the middle of your back. These function as attachment points for various muscles that support each vertebra and the spine, pelvis and head.

The non-sacral vertebrae can be grouped into three sections. Directly above the sacrum is the **lumbar spine** which consists of five very chunky vertebrae that can flex easily forwards, backwards and from side to side, but are capable of only limited twisting movements. Above the lumbar spine are the twelve vertebrae of the **thoracic spine** which provide attachment points for the ribs, making them an intrinsic part of the bony structure of the ribcage. Because they have to support the ribcage and the movements of breathing, these vertebrae are capable of only limited movement themselves. Above the thoracic spine are the seven vertebrae of the **cervical spine** which make up the bony structure of our neck, and support the considerable weight of the head. They articulate with each other quite freely allowing the neck to bend in many different directions.

The top two vertebrae of the cervical spine have a unique structure which is designed to facilitate nodding and turning the head. The joint between the topmost one (the **atlas**)

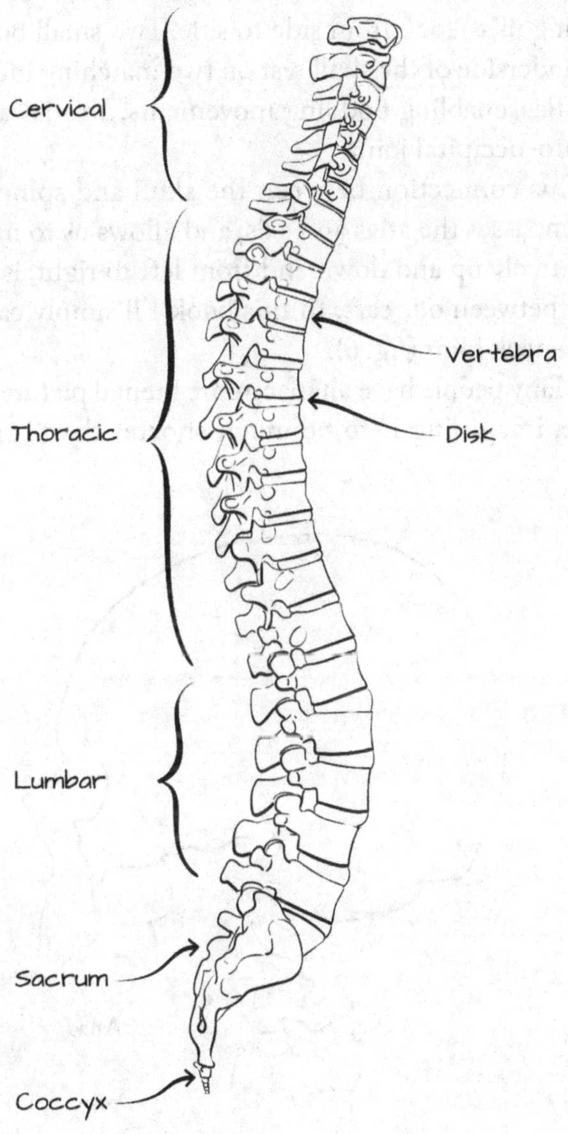

Fig. 5. Parts of the Spine

and the second one down (the **axis**) allows a lot of rotation, helping us to look from side to side. Two small bumps on the underside of the skull rest on two matching indents on the atlas, enabling nodding movements. This is called the **atlanto-occipital** joint.

This connection between the skull and spine, which encompasses the atlas and axis, and allows us to move our head freely up and down and from left to right, is located right between our ears. In this book I'll simply call it the **head–neck joint** (fig. 6).

Many people have an inaccurate mental picture of their spine, imagining it to be much shorter than it is. They

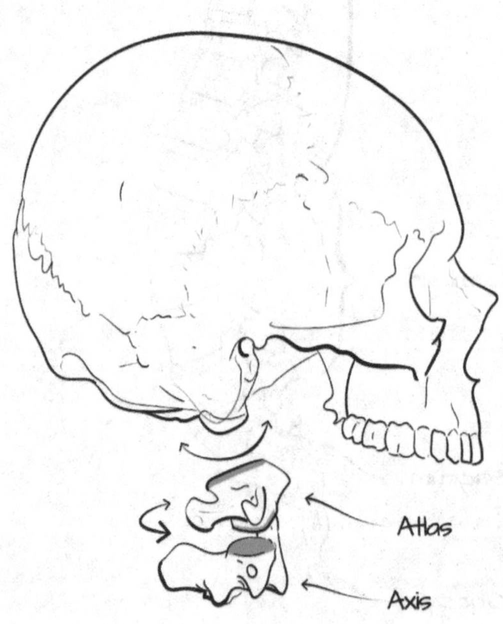

Fig. 6. The Head–Neck Joint

often believe that it runs roughly from the top of their pelvis to the base of their neck. If so, they may be surprised to learn that it actually begins at their coccyx, that it's integrated with their pelvis via the sacrum, and that it finishes much higher than they thought, at their head–neck joint between their ears, creating a single, unified support structure for their torso, neck and head.

The Muscles of the Torso

Three distinct layers of muscle are organised vertically, horizontally and in spiral fashion around the spine, belly, ribcage and neck. Closest to the surface are the **superficial muscles** (fig. 7). These are the ones you can see and feel most easily, such as the pectoral muscles that move the arms and the rectus abdominis, or 'six pack' muscle. They're predominantly used for movement, especially movements of the limbs and head, and are relatively large and powerful.

Arranged in a layer beneath the superficial muscles are the **intermediate muscles** (fig. 8), many of which are also orientated towards movement—especially movements of the torso itself, enabling it to twist and bend forwards and back and from side to side. Many of them also play important roles in breathing, such as the intercostal muscles which run diagonally between each rib, helping to lift them as we breathe in and pulling them down again if we need to exhale forcefully.

The deepest muscles of the torso are the **deep** or **intrinsic** muscles. These are best adapted for stabilisation and support—particularly of the spine, pelvis and head. When everything is working as it should, this leaves the intermediate and superficial muscles free for their primary roles of facilitating movement and breathing (fig. 9).

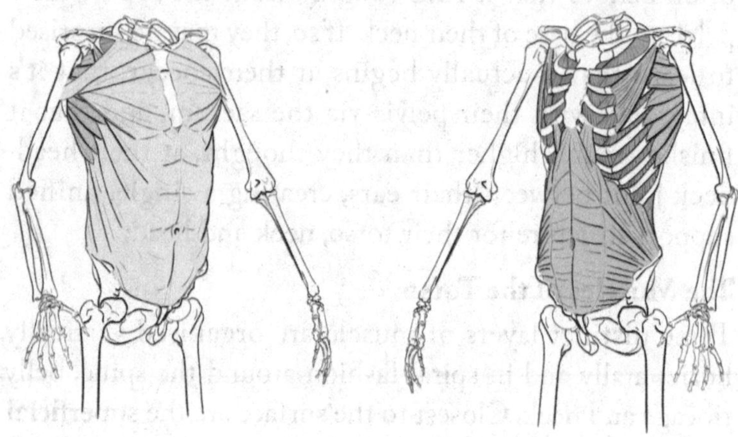

Fig. 7. Superficial Muscles
of the Torso

Fig. 8. Intermediate Muscles
of the Torso

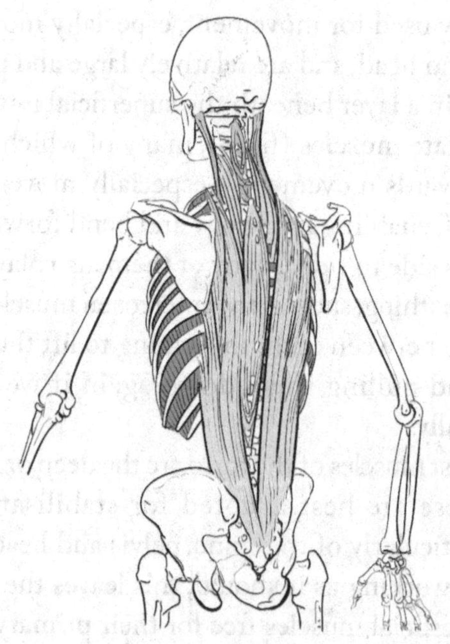

Fig. 9. Deep Muscles of the Spine and Back

The Limbs

Our arms and legs are each formed of three long bones that articulate with each other in various ways to allow the limb as a whole to engage in a wide range of extending, pushing, yielding, supporting, turning and grasping movements (fig. 10). The fingers and toes are made up of a further series of long bones, giving us the ability to grasp with our hands and contact the ground sensitively and flexibly with our feet. Between the fingers and wrist joints, and the toes and ankle joints, are some small, squarish bones (called the carpals and tarsals respectively) that form the heel of the hand and the mid-part of the foot, enabling flexibility and shock absorption. The foot also has a large dedicated heel bone called the calcaneus.

The Pelvis and Shoulder Girdle

The pelvis forms a bony bowl which supports and protects our lower abdominal organs. On each side of the base of the pelvis are two rocker-shaped bones, colloquially known as 'sitting bones' (fig. 4). These bear our weight when we're sitting. You can feel them if you sit on your hands and move around a little.

The legs are attached to the torso via ball-and-socket joints with the pelvis. The arms are attached to the torso less directly via the shoulder blades, and then the collarbones, which together make up the **shoulder girdle** (fig. 4). The collarbones meet the torso at the top of the breastbone. These delicate joints are the only direct, bone-to-bone link between the arms and the torso.

The shoulder blades rest on the back of the ribcage and are held and moved by a web of muscles which attach to various points on the spine, ribcage, and head (fig. 11). These many muscular connections distribute the weight of the arm widely, allowing the shoulder girdle and arm to be supported all day without apparent effort.

The ball-and-socket joint between the arm and shoulder blade has quite a wide range of movement on its own, but this range is increased further because the socket is part

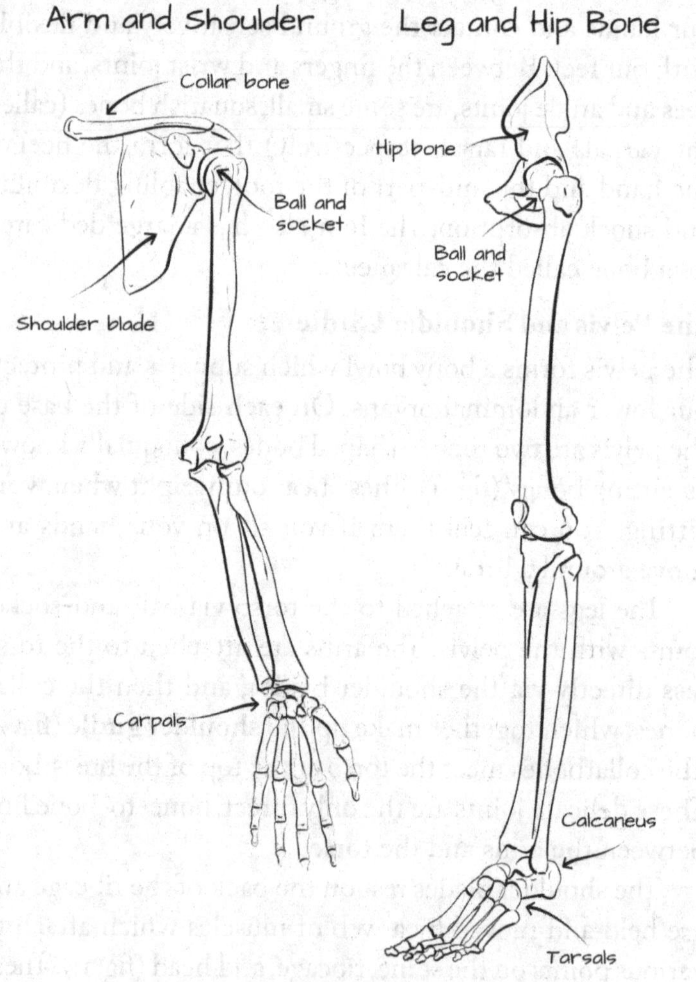

Fig. 10. Bones of the Arms and Legs

of the shoulder blade which can *itself* move in different directions. This enables a much wider range of arm movements than would be possible with the ball-and-socket joint on its own (fig. 12). Without this arrangement, for example, it would be impossible for us to reach up high above our heads or a long way behind or in front of us.

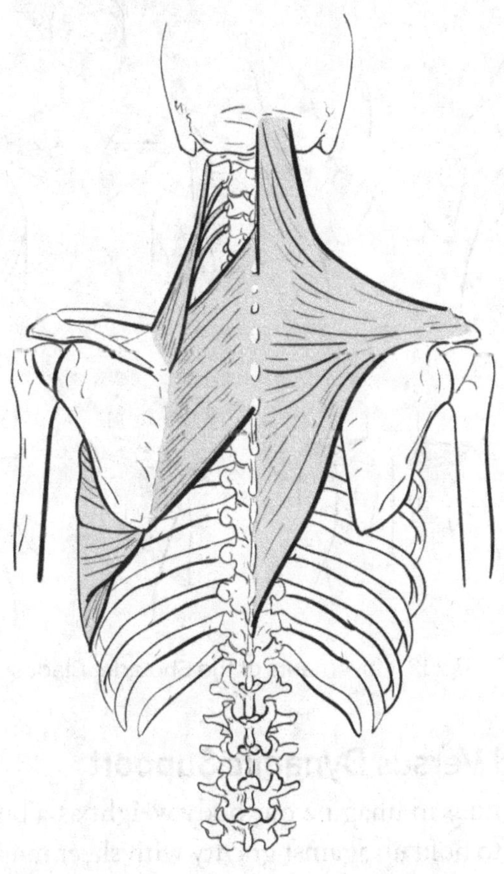

Fig. 11. Muscles of the Shoulder Blades

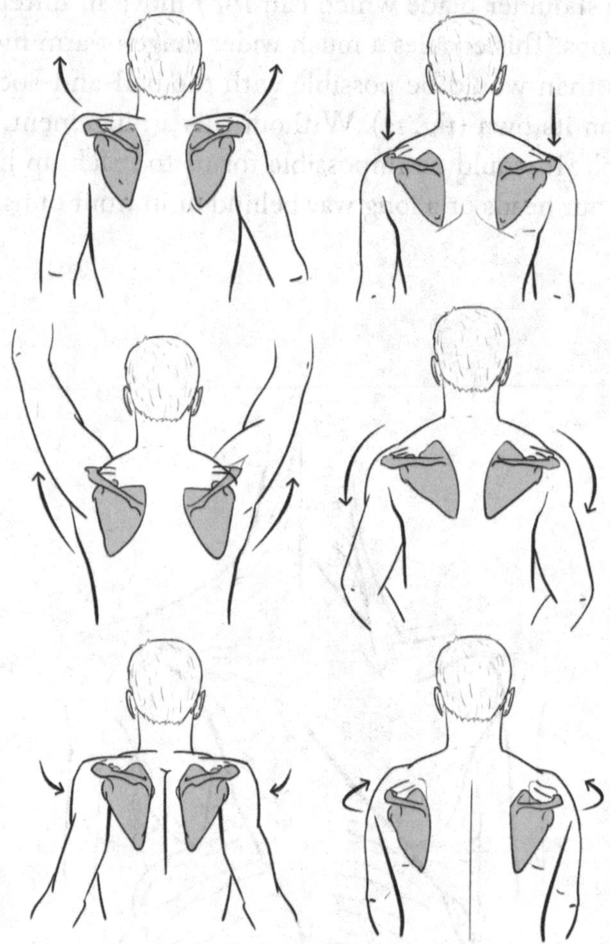

Fig. 12. Movements of the Shoulder Blades

Braced Versus Dynamic Support

It's tempting to imagine our body weight as a burden that we have to hold up against gravity with sheer muscle power and drag around with us wherever we go. But while our muscles *do* play a vital role in supporting us against gravity, they don't generally need to support anything like our entire body weight because most of it is transferred from bone to bone down to the ground. Although some muscle tone is needed to stabilise our joints, when things are working as they should we can rest easily, letting our weight be supported not by our muscles but by the Earth beneath our feet. From this perspective, we can think of ourselves as a flexible, breathing, articulated *stack*.

Paradoxically, our body weight is the key that enables our muscles to work together to dynamically stabilise our structure. Whatever parts of us are in contact with the ground and bearing our weight (our feet when we're standing, our sitting bones when we're sitting, our hands and knees when we're on all fours) are *planted* there by that weight, allowing a chain of muscular stabilisation to activate up from those points of contact through each load-bearing joint of our structure. When we're standing, this ascending chain of support travels from our feet and ankles right up to the head–neck joint at the top of our spine.

Ideally our system organises this chain of muscular support dynamically. This is facilitated by the way our weight is distributed in relation to our main load-bearing joints. The head's centre of gravity, for example, is a little forward of the head–neck joint. Likewise, the torso's centre of gravity is a little in front of the hip joint, and the centre of gravity of the body as a whole is forward of the ankle joint. Because of this, when we are standing our head, torso, and body as a whole all want to gently fall forwards (fig. 13).

This forward tendency enables our head, pelvis and spine to be supported predominantly by dynamic tone in the deep muscles at the back of us, leaving our superficial and intermediate muscles free for movement and breathing.

When all this is working as it should, it's almost as if we're delicately suspended in the Earth's gravitational field—a little like the roadway of a suspension bridge is held floating in space by its towers and cables (fig. 14).

Unfortunately, though, many of us have lost the ability to allow ourselves to be dynamically supported like this. Instead, we get into the habit of rigidly bracing our structure

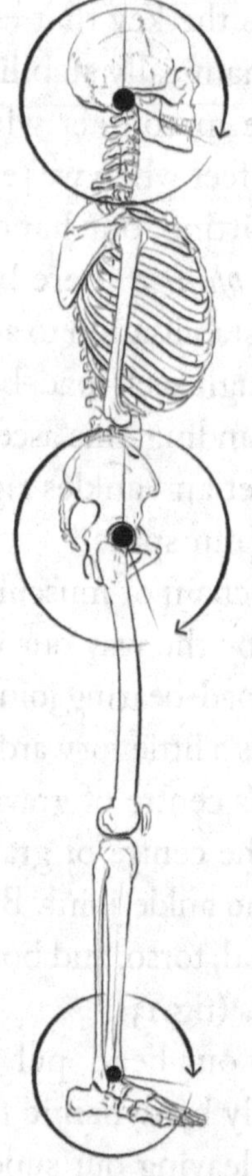

Fig. 13. Tendency
to Fall Forwards

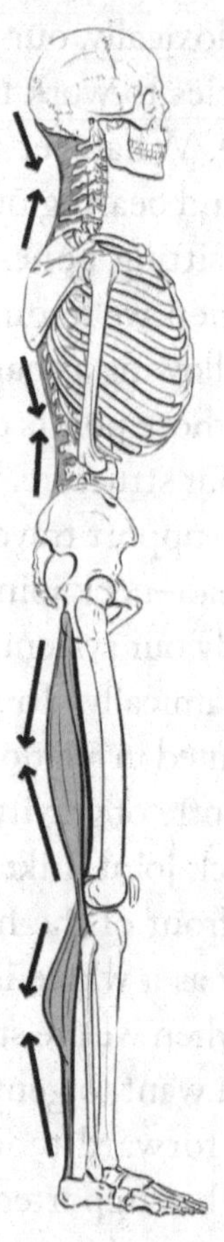

Fig. 14. Support
From the Back

to stay upright, contracting muscles at the front and back of us against each other—including powerful superficial muscles that are optimised for movement rather than support. All this excess muscular tension binds the potentially sensitive, flexible, freely breathing structure of our torso, neck and shoulder girdle into a rigid mass, contracting and compressing our spine and pulling our head back and down onto our shoulders. Ultimately we may get worn out by all this effort and give up the attempt to support ourselves, collapsing instead into an inadequately supported slump.

Chapter Eight
Balance

Whether our structure is being stabilised easily and dynamically or through bracing and excess muscular tension, we'll still fall over if we're not in balance.

Our balance depends on the relationship between our **centre of gravity** and our **base of support**. The centre of gravity is a theoretical point around which the mass of an object is evenly distributed, and on which the force of gravity acts. If we were a perfect sphere it would be right in the centre of us. For an adult who is standing or walking, the centre of gravity is roughly in the middle of the body about ten centimetres below the navel. Its position changes according to the movements we make and the shapes we adopt from moment to moment. Sometimes it can even appear to be completely outside the body.

The base of support is the area of the surface beneath us that includes every part of our body that is in contact with it and bearing our weight (fig. 15). For example, when we're standing, our base of support is the area covered by our feet, together with the area in between them. If we're on all fours it's the area covered by our hands and knees, plus the area between those. So long as we're stationary (or moving slowly enough for momentum and inertia not to be a significant factor), all that's needed for us to stay in balance is for our centre of gravity to be placed somewhere directly above our base of support.

While this is a technically correct way to talk about balance, we can also think about it in a more everyday way, in terms of where our *weight* is. You can feel your weight moving about if you stand and sway gently forwards, backwards and from side to side noticing the changing distribution of pressure on your feet. So long as your weight is placed within the area of your base of support you're in balance and won't fall over.

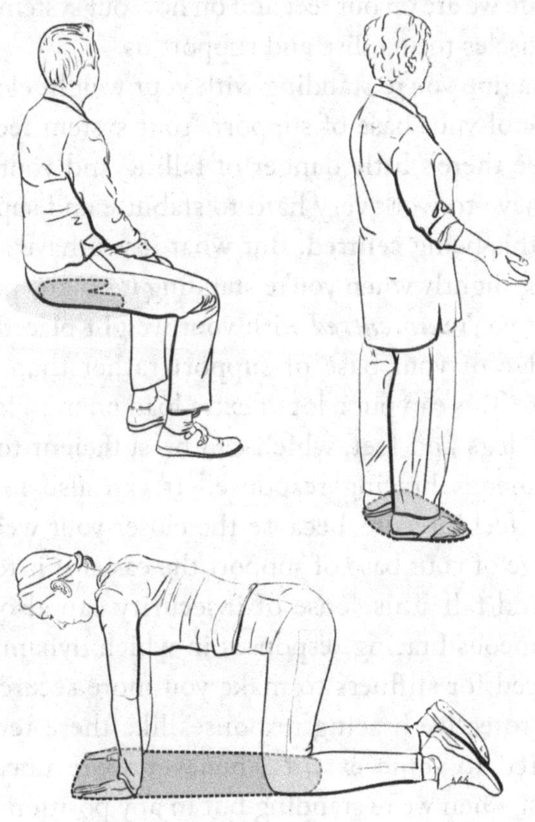

Fig. 15. The Base of Support

Centred and Uncentred Balance

We all seem to understand balance intuitively. We know implicitly that we need to keep our weight within our base of support, and we do it as a matter of course without thinking about it. But we can also think about balance in a more nuanced way by wondering how close our weight is to the *centre* of our base of support at any given moment. This is important because it has a significant impact on how safe we are on our feet and on how our system activates our muscles to stabilise and support us.

Imagine you're standing with your weight close to the middle of your base of support. Your system feels secure because there's little danger of falling and your muscles don't have to work very hard to stabilise and support you. I call this being **centred**. But what if you have a habit of leaning slightly when you're standing (as many people do) so that you're **uncentred** with your weight placed towards the edge of your base of support rather than near the middle? This can put a lot of extra load on muscles in your ankles, legs and feet, which can be sufficient to evoke a spontaneous bracing response.[*] It can also make your system feel insecure, because the closer your weight is to the edge of your base of support the easier it is to overbalance and fall. This sense of insecurity can also activate spontaneous bracing responses in which dynamic ease is sacrificed for stiffness to make you more secure on your feet. Protective bracing responses like these tend to get triggered to some extent whenever we're uncentred—not just when we're standing but in any position in which we're in an active relationship with gravity.

---

[*] See the list of spontaneous bracing strategies on page 42

Momentum and Inertia

So far I've been able to tell a simple story about balance because the examples I've used have assumed we haven't been moving about. But things become a little more complex when we start to move, because of the effects of momentum and inertia.

Momentum is the tendency of a moving body to *keep* moving. If we throw a ball, its momentum keeps it flying towards its destination. Inertia is related to momentum. It's an object's resistance to a change in its state of motion. Think of driving off in a car. We have to start in a low gear because it takes a lot of force to overcome the car's inertia and get it going. Once it's going, it takes a lot of force to overcome its momentum to make it slow down and stop.

When we're moving fairly slowly, the effects of momentum and inertia are so small that they don't noticeably affect us. If I'm doing slow tai chi exercises, for example, then so long as I keep my weight within the area of my base of support I'll remain in balance and won't fall over. Technically this is known as **quasistatic motion** because things still work as if we were standing still.

Once we start to move faster, though, momentum and inertia need to be taken into account. Think about standing on a bus. As it moves off, our body's inertia will make it lag behind the bus so that unless we lean forwards to compensate, we'll fall over backwards. It feels as if the direction of gravity has momentarily tilted forwards, and so we must lean forwards to match it if we're to stay standing as the bus gets up to speed.

As the bus slows, the opposite happens. Momentum makes our body want to continue moving forwards even though the bus is slowing down. It feels as if the direction of gravity has momentarily tilted backwards, so we need to lean backwards to stay standing as the bus comes to a stop. Something similar happens if we set off briskly into a run. Our inertia will make our torso want to lag behind our legs, forcing us to lean forwards as we get going. Conversely, if we're running and we want to stop quickly, we'll need to momentarily lean back a little to counteract our torso's tendency to keep going and overtake our feet.

Of course, the direction of gravity wasn't *really* changing in the above example—it just seemed to be. But thinking about momentum and inertia in terms of their effects on the apparent direction of gravity can be helpful. It allows us to use the same simple understanding of balance (that we must keep our weight within the area of our base of support) not only when we're stationary or moving slowly, but also when we're moving fast enough for momentum and inertia to affect us.

Spontaneous Balance Systems

Many systems in the body help us to stay in balance, and both voluntary and spontaneous processes are involved. Balancing begins, for example, by voluntarily moving ourselves into positions in which our weight is placed within our base of support. Once it's there, though, it needs to stay there. Because of our precarious two-legged stance and complex articulated structure, this requires continuous sensitive adjustments in muscle tone and slight shifts in weight—and the subtlety and speed with which these adjustments need to happen are beyond our ability to control voluntarily. Fortunately, the body has spontaneous systems to help us. These can be divided into two groups.

There are the **equilibrium responses**, which work from the bottom up, shifting our weight in relation to our base of support by making small movements of our pelvis and legs or altering our base of support by moving our feet. And there are the **righting reactions** which work from the top down, using reflexes to alter our centre of gravity by moving our head.

We already came across some of the righting reactions in Chapter Five where we saw that they help stabilise our visual field by keeping our head level as we move about. These reactions are crucial for balance too. Because the head is quite heavy (around five kilograms), it only needs to move slightly to bring about significant shifts in our centre of gravity. Having it automatically kept level and stable rather than wobbling around is a big help in staying in balance. In addition, if our body starts tipping away from vertical, reflexes tilt our head in the opposite direction using its weight to help us return to uprightness.

These righting reactions are based on fairly simple reflex-based mechanisms. The equilibrium responses, on the other hand, work in a more complex way. If we drift just slightly out of balance, small, spontaneous movements of our ankle joints, hips and pelvis will shift our centre of gravity back over our feet. The more serious the disturbance, the more robust these movements become. If our system detects that we're an imminent danger of falling, they can become very robust indeed. Our arms may rise spontaneously to give us greater control. We might even find ourselves taking an involuntary step to one side or forwards or backwards as our system tries to keep our base of support beneath us. In extreme cases, our feet spontaneously move apart and our knees bend, increasing our stability by lowering our centre of gravity while our arms get thrown out like a tightrope walker. All this happens in a moment without a deliberate decision on our part.

Dynamic Balance

Not falling over is so important that our system will do whatever it can to prevent it. The systems involved are highly resilient and will usually work well enough to keep us upright regardless of whether we're being stabilised and supported by muscular bracing or in an easy, dynamic way. The more dynamic our musculature is, though, the better our balance system works, and the more subtlety and nuance it can bring to balancing us because our body is freer to move and respond sensitively as needed, while our system receives richer sensory information from our continuously adjusting muscles and wide peripheral vision.

We become more aware of the importance of dynamic stabilisation and support for balance when doing demanding activities like walking on a tightrope or slackline. If you try this and you're not used to it, you'll most likely find that your nervousness at the thought of falling will make your muscles spontaneously brace and tighten as soon as you step onto the line. If you persevere, though, you may discover that this muscular bracing—though it may feel safer to begin with—is the last thing you need, limiting the freedom with which your system can respond from moment to moment and making it much more likely you'll fall. To balance easily and securely we need to learn to trust and *let go*, choosing not to tighten up defensively or to over-control, giving our system's spontaneous responses the best possible chance to help us.

Chapter Nine
Movement

To do anything useful in the world we must be able to voluntarily control our actions, asking our body to move in ways that conform to our intentions. But these voluntary actions still require a lot of help from lower-level, spontaneous parts of our nervous system.

Because our skeleton is an articulated structure consisting of many rigid parts, even simple actions involve the interaction of several joints. To reach out and pick something up, for example, requires coordinated movements of numerous joints in our shoulder, arm and wrist, together with simultaneous coordination of joints in our hand and fingers. But despite the underlying complexity, these elaborate compound movements seem quite simple and straightforward to perform. When we reach out with our hand, we don't have to think about our elbow, shoulder joint, wrist or all the ways our fingers can move—we can think of the movement as a single action. We can have a broad intention, and our neuromuscular system takes care of many of the details for us. This works not just with the hands but with any part of our body. We can move our foot through space, or our elbow, or our pelvis, or we can ask our shoulder girdle to rotate, or our head to turn to look behind us, and generally our system will sort out the necessary movements of the various joints involved without us having to control them all individually.

The ability of the brain and nervous system to organise complex, multi-joint coordinations like this is extremely sophisticated. We can even act as if tools we are using are extensions of ourselves. If I'm hammering a nail, for example, I can direct the hammer by thinking about its head moving through space as if it were a part of me. I don't need to think about moving my body directly at all. Somehow my system sorts out the underlying coordination implied by my general intentions.

Many things come together to make complex movement possible. All animals, for example, have access to innate, inborn movement patterns called **motor programmes**. Reaching, grasping and standing movements are examples of these. Even babies seem to understand implicitly that their hands are there to enable them to reach and grasp. They don't need to be taught this: they have the wish to reach for something and the movement happens automatically.

Motor programmes are assisted by the fact that certain muscles and muscle groups are wired so that a single nerve impulse can move them all at once. These interconnections are known as **synergies**. Try holding your arm extended with your palm facing upwards then slowly bending your wrist and elbow simultaneously towards you. Generally, this feels quite easy and natural to do. However, if you hold your arm extended with your palm upwards but this time, while you bend your elbow towards you, you simultaneously bend your hand *away* from you at the wrist, it generally feels rather awkward and unnatural. The first attempt felt easier because the muscles that bend the elbow and wrist towards us are synergistically connected. These kinds of neuromuscular connections facilitate and guide many of our characteristic movements.

We get additional help for activities that require predictable, repetitive movements from small clusters of nerve cells in the spinal column called **central pattern generators**. These tiny, low-level neural circuits generate the basic patterns of muscle activation needed for activities such as walking, running, swimming, breathing, chewing, swallowing and so on. We can voluntarily modify these as needed (perhaps taking an extra big step while we're walking to avoid a puddle), but the basic underlying patterns are innate.

Everything Connects

As we move and take action in the world, motor programmes, pattern generators, muscle synergies and other movement mechanisms combine, interacting with our systems for attention, emotional arousal, stabilisation, balance and support in complex ways that can foster either ease and skilfulness or bracing, awkwardness and stress. It's a deeply integrated system. Parts influence other parts and are influenced back in turn. Everything connects.

As we go on, I'll be asking how our voluntary actions can work in harmony with this extraordinary integrated system, and how we can encourage the functions we've been talking about to organise healthily together so that whatever we're up to—whether it's as challenging as playing sports or a musical instrument or as simple as going for a walk or washing the dishes—we can do it with a renewed sense of ease, freedom and skill.

Part Two
Fundamentals of Skill

Chapter Ten
The Adaptable Self

An important difference between ourselves and other animals is that their behaviour is more instinctive and predetermined than ours. They're equipped from birth with a comprehensive set of innate abilities which appear as they develop and grow without having to be figured out and learned through thought and reason. If a dog is raised by humans without ever seeing another member of its species it will end up walking and running like any other dog. It doesn't have to be shown how to do it. But human children who have been abandoned and adopted and raised by dogs from a young age don't generally learn to walk upright on their own—they tend to end up walking on all fours, like a dog. Similarly, a dog will learn to feed itself in the usual canine fashion without having to be shown how, but for human children to learn to eat like adults requires practice and the help and example of others. So although we have similar spontaneous systems to other animals, we have to go through a much longer and more conscious process to mature and learn how to use them. A large part of the 'instruction set' for being a human is therefore held not in our genes but in our *culture*. It's shared and passed on by teaching and modelling rather than inherited directly. To use a contemporary analogy, compared to other animals we're more software and less hardware.

Although our developmental process as children is slow and laborious, it has significant advantages. If locomotion, for example, developed as automatically for us as it does for other animals, we'd be stuck with a few particular ways of doing it. We could choose between some characteristic gaits—walking, trotting, running—and that would be the limit of our capabilities. But because our development is less fixed, we're free to develop numerous variations on the theme. Hopping, skipping, dancing, ice-skating, speed-walking, skateboarding, cycling—all this is possible because we can make detailed and reasoned choices about how to use our legs to get about. Pigs can't rebel against their instincts and decide to move like antelopes. But we can choose from an infinite number of ways to move. If you decided to move like an antelope you could probably have a good go at it! Uniquely among animals, we can endlessly expand the possibilities open to us through inventing, learning, perfecting and passing on new skills.

Controlling Ourselves

Our ability to develop, transmit and learn new skills depends on us having a high degree of conscious control over ourselves. In particular, we need to be able to make our bodies move in ways that conform to our ideas and intentions, to direct our attention to where it's needed, and to have a degree of control over our emotional responses.

Controlling Movement

We humans have an unusually refined ability to voluntarily control our movements. Other animals can move their bodies voluntarily too, but what is unusual about us is how *much* we can do this—isolating this part from that and getting them to work separately and together as we see fit. We can move each joint of our body within its entire range of movement, one at a time or in combination with others. We can voluntarily and deliberately stiffen individual joints or relax them at will. And, as we've seen, we can even override our autonomic nervous system and control our breathing—speeding it up, slowing it down, or making it deeper and shallower in any way we like.

Think about a complex task like learning to play the violin. Just holding the instrument and making the movements needed to produce sound from it is excruciatingly difficult and awkward to begin with. To become proficient we need to go through an intricate conscious process, practising numerous precise, unintuitive movements that have no parallel in nature until we can draw on them instantly, with phenomenal accuracy, to produce the sounds we want. No other animal is capable of anything remotely approaching this.

Directing the Attention

In addition to this refined ability to control our movements, we also need to be able to voluntarily and precisely direct our attention. We've seen that complex human skills require many shifts of attention from one aspect of the activity to another while keeping a global awareness of ourselves and the space around us. Learning a complex skill often requires us to *deliberately* manage these attention shifts to begin with, noticing what we need to pay attention to and when, until doing so becomes an integrated part of the activity.

Regulating Emotional Responses

As well as voluntarily controlling our movements and directing our attention, we often also need to consciously influence our emotional states—particularly potentially disruptive high-arousal ones like fear, anxiety and excitement. This is an essential ability, allowing us to perform complex tasks in circumstances which evolution could never have prepared us for. We have no instincts, for example, to help us with situations like dealing with an angry boss, facing a large audience who expect us to entertain them, or driving on a motorway with huge trucks thundering past in the rain. Without the ability to regulate our emotions, such arousing and threatening situations would likely result in us being overwhelmed by primitive defensive responses causing us to lash out, flee or freeze, none of which would likely serve us well under the circumstances!

There are several ways we can regulate our emotions. One way is to change the way we think about what we're experiencing. We might reframe a scary situation as exciting, rationally consider whether our fears are valid, or look for the positives in a negative situation. But we can also regulate our emotions *physically* through the body or by seeking out supportive contact and connection with others.

Regulating Through the Body

We've seen how, when our limbic brain detects a potential threat, it activates the sympathetic nervous system to prepare us to fight, flee or freeze. Our muscles brace and tighten, our field of attention narrows and fixes, and our breathing becomes faster and shallower, shifting higher up in the ribcage. This relationship between anxiety and the body is intriguing because to some extent it works both ways. Anxiety affects the body but it's also possible for us to influence our musculature, breath and attention to reverse those effects—gently asking our attention to expand and soften, our braced joints to let go, and our breathing to release. This can help to create feelings in the body associated with comfort and safety, activating the parasympathetic nervous system so that our system settles and quietens down again.*

Regulating Through Social Connection

We can also calm and regulate our emotions through supportive contact with others. Our bodies and nervous systems are continuously responding to each other—attuning, connecting and disconnecting through posture, mirroring, eye contact and many other mechanisms. This makes it easy to 'catch' both positive and negative moods and emotions from those around us. If we're surrounded by angry, stressed people, for example, it's difficult to stay calm ourselves. Conversely, the soothing words, eye contact and supportive touch of a concerned friend or relative can help us calm down and return to balance. Intriguingly, many of the organs that help us form and maintain social relationships and connect with others—such as the muscles that control our facial expression, eyes and voice, and even the tiny muscles in the inner ear which help us tune in to the frequencies of speech—are innervated by nerves linked to the calming parasympathetic nervous system. It seems we're literally hardwired to gain support from others and to help each other regulate our emotions.

Knowing What to Do

While it's essential to be able to consciously control our movements and attention, and to influence our emotional states, if we want to apply these abilities to help us learn

---

* ...so long as certain pitfalls are avoided which we'll talk about later.

new skills, we also need to understand ourselves and the world around us. Broadly speaking, there are two ways we can do this. We can do so in a linear, time-based way in terms of cause and effect, which I'll call **procedural understanding**, or in an intuitive, all-of-a-piece way in which our situation is seen, understood and responded to as a whole, in the moment, which I'll call **tacit understanding**.

Procedural Understanding

Think for a moment about the process of learning some new skill. Whether it's as simple as a child taking its first steps or as complex as learning the violin, we originally conceive it as a whole thing. We imagine playing beautiful music or crossing the room on our own two feet. How lovely that will be! But, as soon as we start trying to learn, it can all seem rather difficult and confusing. There's a gulf between where we are and where we want to be. To begin with we have to go through a process of grappling with the problem, trying to get a handle on what we're doing. We must start humbly, breaking things down into more manageable parts before combining them into the living, breathing whole we first imagined. A pole-vaulter needs to know how to hold the pole, where and when to place it and the best way to coordinate their movements to get themselves over the bar. A violinist needs to know how to hold the instrument, how to read music, where to place their fingers on the strings and so on. We can't even stand up, feed ourselves with a fork or walk across the room without having first developed an objective understanding of the steps required to do so—even if these were learned so long ago that they've come to feel completely natural and inevitable.

This objective, linear, this-follows-that appreciation of an activity can be either conscious or subconscious. Think about helping someone learn to ride a bike. There are various instructions you could give them: 'Sit on the saddle with a leg on each side; hold the handlebars and apply the brakes; set the pedals so that one is just forward of top dead centre; put your foot on the top pedal, push down on it and release the brakes; if you think you're going to fall put on the brakes and put your foot down', and so on.

When you have this kind of understanding of the order and sequence of actions necessary to carry out a task, and you can put them into words to communicate them to yourself and others, it's called **explicit** knowledge.

But what if you learned to ride a bike as a child but you never articulated it to yourself anything like as clearly as I did just now. Perhaps you just watched what the other children were up to and threw yourself into it repeatedly until you got the hang of it. Even if this was the case, I bet when you read my list of instructions above you recognised it, or something very like it. This indicates that you have **implicit** knowledge of how to ride a bike.[*] For our purposes, implicit knowledge is when you know what to do but haven't clearly articulated that knowledge to yourself in words yet. But you *could* articulate it if you wanted to and thought about it for a bit.

Implicit and explicit knowledge are both forms of procedural understanding. They're similar in that each involves appreciating ourselves and the world in an objective way, mentally splitting reality into parts and deciding what to

---

[*] Note that I am borrowing the words 'procedural', 'explicit', 'implicit' and 'tacit' from knowledge theory and not everyone in the field uses them in exactly the same way.

do in terms of how those parts move and relate to each other through time and space. But while this way of understanding things is essential, it's not sufficient to enable us to become proficient in new skills. For that, tacit understanding is needed too.

Tacit Understanding

Think about riding a bike again. We know that to make it go we have to sit on the saddle, hold the handlebars and turn the pedals. We know we can steer by turning the handlebars left and right. But, even knowing this, when we first learn to ride a bike there's a period of trial and error when the task seems quite impossible. There's so much to coordinate simultaneously and everything we do seems to affect everything else. When we shift our balance to try and stay on we turn sideways into a bush. Turning the pedals moves our weight around in unexpected ways, and going downhill and uphill feel impossibly different to each other. When we lean it affects the steering, and when we steer it makes us lean. To top it all, staying on is harder when we're going slowly (which feels safer) and easier when we're going fast (which feels dangerous)!

What's missing is a visceral, *embodied* understanding of the situation. To begin with we don't know how hard we need to push off to get going, or how big a shift in weight or steering is needed to correct for disturbances in balance, or what any of that feels like. We can't judge when and how hard to apply the brakes, or how to turn the pedals without destabilising ourselves. And because the situation is fluid and constantly changing there can be no foolproof formula to help us anyway. But, nevertheless, with practice, gradually or quite suddenly, we begin to get the hang of it.

We find we can balance ourselves and judge the constantly changing forces involved as we zoom along. We begin to intuitively understand the dynamic relationships between weight, balance and momentum in an immediate, in-the-moment sort of way. Not only do we understand that we need to shift our weight as we push off, but we know that we need to do it 'just so'. We feel ourselves tipping to one side and intuitively know the timing and strength of the tiny shift in steering needed to bring the bike beneath us again, in the moment, all-of-a-piece.

One of the features of tacit understanding is that it can't be put precisely into words. We can hint at aspects of it by describing qualities of the experience (faster, slower, gently, firmly, expansively, delicately and so on), but we can't transfer the knowledge we have directly to another person through language or diagrams. No one can tell you how to ride a bike, play a violin or pole-vault in a way that enables you to go straight out and do it. A good teacher can give you plenty of pointers, but there's always a gulf between the description and the act itself.

Tacit and procedural understanding are very different, but each is essential. They go together hand in hand. To do any task well we have to understand the order and sequence of things *and* know what's required in our bodies through practice and experience. We must be comfortable thinking about the activity and refining our mental understanding of it while realising that it can never be fully captured that way—it can only really be known in the moment.

Chapter Eleven

Action Sequences and Habits

Our ability to understand ourselves and the world around us, to reason and make decisions, and to voluntarily control our movements, attention and emotional arousal makes it possible for us to learn new skills and deal with novel situations that evolution didn't prepare us for. But this still wouldn't be much use if we had to deliberately control every detail each time we did a particular task. Imagine if whenever you arrived home you had to remember how to use the lock—how to raise the key and insert it, which way to turn it and the necessary coordination of your fingers and wrist. Or think how tiresome it would be if every time you ate you had to carefully and deliberately guide the food from the plate into your mouth as if you were still two years old. Fortunately, though, as well as having the ability to think, reason and move our bodies, we can also store and recall useful patterns and sequences of movements by developing **action sequences** and **habits**.

Action Sequences

An action sequence is a chain of movements that is learned and refined by being repeated over and over again. The more we repeat it the easier it gets, the faster we can do it and the less thought and mental effort we have to give to it. Through repetition, the actions become physically wired into neurones in our brain in a process known as neuroplasticity.

Even simple activities, like standing up or walking, initially require us to learn sequences of movements that enable us to do them fluidly and easily without having to figure everything out from scratch each time. The more complex an activity, the more sequences we need to learn so that we can respond appropriately to a wider and wider range of contingencies in a wider and wider range of circumstances. This is one reason why perfecting a demanding skill like playing a musical instrument takes so many years of work. Huge numbers of action sequences have to be practised and refined over and over until they become reliably available to us whenever they're needed.

Action sequences can be complex and subtle, and involve numerous steps, including ones to do with shifts of attention and regulating emotional arousal. A skilled violinist, for example, may go through a sequence before beginning to play that includes lifting the instrument and placing it just so, orienting themselves to the space around them, letting go of any breath-holding or other unnecessary muscular tension, refocusing their attention on the instrument and the music, and raising the bow. All of this can happen in a few moments as they prepare to play in a structured, intelligent way.

Action sequences have a degree of flexibility about them. Having learned to drive, for example, I can choose to change gears in a precise, snappy way or a relaxed, lackadaisical way. In either case I don't have to think about what I'm doing in detail—I can draw on the same underlying pattern of movements I originally learned. Similarly, when a skilled violinist plays a musical pattern that they know well, they don't always have to play it with the same phrasing, or at the same speed or tempo. They can play the pattern in many different ways, even shifting from one way to another in the middle.

When we use action sequences, we can be conscious of them right the way through, staying mentally present at each step. But when a sequence is well learned, we can also allow it to continue to unfold on its own once we've initiated it while we focus on some other aspect of the activity.

Think about learning to drive a car. To begin with it can feel overwhelming to remember all the different tasks and sub-tasks involved and the order they come in. Because of this, a good driving instructor will help you to build up the skill bit by bit, starting from the basics like adjusting the seat and the mirrors before going on to the practical side of actually making the car go—working the gears, brakes and steering and so on. Gradually these simple tasks become so well learned that most of the time we no longer need to focus on them, leaving us free to think about where we're headed and how to interact with other road users. Pulling out of a junction on a dark and rainy night, we can put most of our attention on the traffic and the road ahead rather than on the movements needed to grasp the gear-stick, select the right gear, find the biting point of the clutch and release the brakes.

Healthy and Unhealthy Action Sequences

Just because an action sequence gets the job done at a practical level doesn't mean it's good for us. Healthy action sequences work in harmony with our body's spontaneous systems for sensing, stabilisation, support and balance to enable freedom and ease in the activity. Less healthy ones work *against* those systems, triggering bracing and tightness in our bodies and unnecessary awkwardness in our actions, even if they still give us a basic level of competence. Perhaps we've unwittingly learned action sequences in which we concentrate and over-focus our attention, or that uncentre us causing our muscles to spontaneously brace and tighten. Or maybe we've practised sequences that demand excessive muscular effort. In time, an accumulation of these kinds of unhealthy action sequences can end up creating bracing, excess tension and effortfulness in almost everything we do.

Habit

Action sequences begin with a *choice*. I choose to get out of my chair, or to play a C major scale on the piano, or to change gear in my car. But there's another type of learned movement sequence that happens unconsciously, without a choice, which we call habits. Habits are action sequences that have become automatic, so they get triggered without our conscious choice or awareness. They form when we repeatedly do the same thing in the same context and are rewarded in some way for doing so. The reward can be external, such as getting some kind of treat, or internal, such as a feeling of accomplishment, pride, acceptance or safety. It's like training a puppy. If you keep getting him to sit down while saying the word 'sit' and then give him a treat, in the end the behaviour becomes so ingrained that he responds to 'sit' even if you don't give him the treat afterwards.

This is a key feature of a habit: the behaviour pattern has become detached both from our conscious intentions *and* from the reward we get from doing it. Only the trigger is needed for it to unfold automatically with no regard for the consequences. If I walk past the biscuit jar, wonder whether I'd like one, ponder how many calories I've eaten today, decide that there is room for just a little one, take one and eat it, that is a choice. However, if I wander past, reach out, take a biscuit, and am halfway through it before I have even noticed what I'm up to, that is a habit! I may have already overeaten that day and get no pleasure from eating the biscuit, but the habit gets triggered anyway just by walking past the jar.

The word 'habit' has some negative connotations, but habits can also have a positive aspect. As a young child you don't automatically put on a seat belt when you get in a car. But if every time you get in the car an adult tells you to do so and you are rewarded in some way (perhaps by feeling safer or more grown up or by being praised), in time it becomes a habit. In the end, you climb into the car and put on the seat belt even if you're lost in thought or anxiously worrying about something else. The habit helps to keep you safe. You may go for months getting in your car every day without once consciously registering that you're putting on your seat belt. The same goes for looking both ways before crossing the road, or locking the doors of your home before you go to bed at night.

It's our habits which enable us to walk about, drive or do the washing up while completely lost in our thoughts without needing to give conscious attention to what we're doing. This has a positive side. As humans, we do sometimes need to think deeply about things, and being able to be lost in our thoughts while carrying out essential everyday tasks is useful. But it has downsides too. To move and function at our best, we need some conscious awareness of ourselves, our surroundings and what we're up to. Though habits can get us through the day, they're not sensitive, subtle or fully responsive to the constantly changing circumstances we face from moment to moment. They can work well enough to get the job done—but usually not well enough to get it done with sensitivity, skilfulness and ease.

Often, as we grow older, more and more of our movements and activities become habitual. Simple things such as the way we stand up and sit down, how we move our limbs, the way we hold ourselves and the way we focus our attention or deal with our emotional responses all become more and more unconscious, unfolding without choice or awareness. This is particularly a problem when the action sequences the habits were based on were unhealthy to begin with, putting our body under constant stress and strain as we go about our lives. This can end up with us uncomfortable, in pain and, in the long term, even seriously harming ourselves.

Later on in the book we'll be looking at how we can go back to basics, regaining a healthy awareness of ourselves and the way we do things, unlearning unhealthy action sequences and habits, and discovering helpful new ones that work in harmony with our system, enabling dynamic ease to activate in everything we do.

Chapter Twelve
Circling the Problem

So far in this part of the book I've talked about various aspects of learning, particularly with regard to acquiring concrete physical skills. I've pointed out the extraordinary ability we have to control our movements, attention and emotional arousal compared to other animals. We've explored the difference between procedural and tacit knowledge, and seen how the steps needed to perform complex tasks can be stored in action sequences and habits. But how can we go about bringing these disparate elements together into coherent, competent activity?

One way I like to describe it is that we need to **circle the problem**. We start by working with the most basic elements of the activity—dipping in here, dipping in there, pulling out to see the whole picture before coming in close again to work on this or that part, looking from one angle and then another as each circling of the material slightly deepens and widens our understanding. For example, you could be working on a piece on the violin and decide to pay *particular* attention to your bowing for a while, and then to your left hand, and then to your set-up or your intonation. We engage in the activity while focusing on discrete parts of it that need attention, foregrounding them while allowing the other parts to unfold automatically as well as they are able.

As we improve, the circles get wider. The basics become increasingly secure and taken for granted. We work on more complex aspects of the skill while our growing proficiency gives us the freedom to step back more and more as fragments of understanding begin to spontaneously coalesce into a more integrated whole. We find ourselves beginning to shift from a hesitant, deliberate, laboured focus on details towards being more of a guider–overseer, letting action sequences unfold, skilfully making choices, allowing things to happen on the fly just as they are needed, intervening in the detail only when we see it's necessary to keep things on track.

Many people feel daunted by the thought of learning new things, particularly in the early stages when everything seems so strange and unfamiliar. They may avoid trying to develop skills they'd be quite capable of getting to grips with, believing them to be out of reach. But this is a shame, because we humans are *natural integrators*. We're *inherently* good at pulling fragments of skill and understanding together into living, breathing wholes—so long as we're willing to give the process the necessary time, space and attention. We're *designed* to integrate complexity into simplicity. We *evolved* to do it. We are, in fact, *integrating animals*. We don't have to force it. We just have to agree to consistently be in the process of learning—to think, feel, plan, imagine, experiment, practise, trust and take time. Gradually, in a process beyond words, it happens. Driving the car we find to our surprise that we're thinking about where we're going rather than about how to change gear. Playing the violin we notice suddenly that we're thinking about the flow of the music rather than worrying about where to find the notes on the neck. Bit by bit it feels like we're getting somewhere until, to our delight, we arrive at the simple vision we had right at the beginning. We're no longer struggling with details and how they fit together. The activity is no longer fragmented into parts. It's no longer a struggle. It all becomes very simple and clear. At last we are playing beautiful music, or crossing the room, easily and gracefully, on our own two feet.

Part Three
The Skilful Self

Chapter Thirteen
Being and Doing

It's sometimes suggested that we modern people spend too much time doing and not enough time being. If only we could learn to be less driven and goal-directed—take a bit more time to rest and smell the roses—then perhaps we'd be happier and do less harm to ourselves and others. There is some truth in this! But of course, as humans we also need to be doing stuff. Food doesn't put itself on the table, clothes don't sew themselves, and culture isn't presented ready-made. Everything we have is earned by ourselves or others through learning, application and effort. And yet, no matter what we're up to, we're still always in some state of being, and that state comes with us into our actions and the things that we do.

We saw earlier that, when we think about an activity and consider how we might do it better, we tend to focus on the most obvious aspects of what we're up to. If we're playing the piano we think about moving our fingers and getting the right notes, and perhaps not quite so much about the underlying state of mind we bring to our practice. If we're running, we think about the way we move our arms and legs and about how to build muscle to make those movements stronger, but perhaps less about how the muscular stabilisation that underpins that strength and those movements is organised. If we think about the way we do the washing up we might pay a lot of attention to the physical movements of picking up, scrubbing and putting down the dishes but rather less to whether we're centred and breathing freely and easily as we do so. This excessive focus on the surface elements of what we're doing is unfortunate because the degree of ease and skilfulness we can manifest in our activities depends on the quality of those deeper factors which are always there, for better or worse, under the surface.

We've also seen that even though many of us habitually move and do things in ways that are more awkward than they need to be, and which put our bodies under a lot of stress and strain, our system actually evolved to enable us to move and be supported in a lovely, easy, dynamic way. Ease is our natural state. We're supposed to shift into braced, concentrated, rigid states only briefly—when we want to focus our gaze on something tiny, or need to lift, push or pull very heavy loads, or when our system spontaneously mobilises for self-defence. And ideally we revert to dynamic ease as soon as the need has passed. Ease *wants* to happen. It's our system's innate tendency, and it activates spontaneously whenever the conditions are right.*

One implication of this is that there's a responsibility on 'us'—the voluntary self—to make sure that we're not getting in the way of ease, either through our conscious actions or through unconscious habits that we've built up over time. Everything we do either supports or undermines our system's spontaneous attempts to organise freely and easily from moment to moment. We'll be uncovering more

---

* Sometimes injury or medical conditions can get in the way of this happening. See Appendix B for an explanation of how the principles in this book can still be beneficially applied when this is the case.

about this ongoing interdependent relationship between the voluntary and spontaneous parts of ourselves in this next part of the book.

Chapter Fourteen

Seven Qualities of Ease

Let's pause for a moment, put all the information and ideas we've been looking at to one side, and return to the immediacy of the senses.

Take a moment to gently sigh, or to breathe out slowly. Maybe notice the sensation of the furniture and clothes where they touch your skin, and any feelings and sensations from inside of you, and particularly your breath as it moves gently in and out.

Whereabouts in your body feels good right now?

Even if there is discomfort somewhere in the body, there's always somewhere else that feels at least *somewhat* more comfortable.

What sounds can you hear—perhaps the wind, a clock ticking or the passing traffic? Just be with them for a while. Maybe give yourself permission to put the book down, look around and notice what there is to see all about you, dropping gently into the experience of the moment.

When you're ready, let's go on.

In Part One of the book we were thinking about the Self mostly from a rational, science-like viewpoint as if we were interested observers peering in at ourselves from the outside. We were looking from the perspective of *parts*, breaking the Self into pieces to understand how the bits we observe seem to work and relate to each other. This objective, rational understanding provides us with a helpful foundation to build on. But as we begin to consider things more deeply, we also need to start looking from a more tacit perspective, asking what it's like to *experience* all these systems, structures and processes working together in ourselves. What are they like subjectively, seen from the *inside*?

Imagine if, right now, I could move you magically towards the easy, harmonious end of the continuum of discomfort and ease which we met earlier. What would that be like? Let's assume for the moment that you're not doing anything in particular in this free and easy state, but are just standing or sitting quietly and comfortably, in neutral, with no sense of effort, tension or strain. What sort of qualities might you notice in yourself in such a state?

Here are seven likely possibilities:

1. **Quietness**. There would be a calm quietness in your body and nervous system.

2. **Presence**. You would be *here*, in the moment, rather than tuned out, distracted or lost in mental preoccupation about the past or future.

3. **Openness**. Your field of attention—and particularly your visual field—would be open and free to move, all your senses freely receptive to whatever was happening inside and out.

4. **Freedom**. There would be a sense of unbraced freedom throughout your structure—and particularly in the movements of your breath.

5. **Centredness**. Your weight would be placed delicately, somewhere near the middle of your base of support.

6. **Dynamic Stabilisation.** Your body would be subtly moving and adjusting from moment to moment as it dynamically stabilised you in the field of gravity.

7. **Grounded Support.** You would be in sensitive, dynamic contact with the ground beneath you, enabling a rising chain of dynamic support, leaving your spine free to adopt its full, unforced length and your head to balance freely on top.

If the state of ease that I'm talking about isn't very familiar at the moment then these words—quietness, presence, openness, freedom, centredness, dynamic stabilisation and grounded support—may not mean that much to you yet. You might get a rough idea from the verbal description, but to really understand what I'm talking about you will need to experience them for yourself. Hopefully, in time, you will. You may even come to find your *own* words for these qualities—ones that resonate more deeply for you than mine do. So perhaps it's best for now to treat the ones I'm using simply as helpful signposts. They're *pointing* towards something. There's an interesting journey to go on to get there, but at least the words can give you an idea of the sort of direction it would be sensible to be heading off in. And, just as importantly, they can give you an idea of which way *not* to go. We'll be talking a lot more about this idea of what we *don't* want later on. But, in the meantime, let's look more closely at each of these qualities of ease.

Quietness

What does it mean to be really calm and quiet? I don't mean quiet in the sense of being immobile or inactive, or not talking or making a noise. I mean what is it like to be *internally* calm and quiet, no matter what you're doing externally? This is not the sort of quietness that is associated with being languid or sleepy, nor the intense quietness that comes from the kind of meditation where you still your mind by repeating a mantra or concentrating on a physical sensation or image. Rather, I'm thinking about an *alert* quietness that goes hand in hand with being present and in touch with yourself and your surroundings.

Such quietness doesn't preclude action! A person can be calm and collected even amid a great emergency. Like the quietness of a skilled martial artist, ours can be like the still eye at the heart of a storm.

When our system is quiet, we experience it in both the mind and the body. Even if our mind is active and thinking about this or that, it does so gently and spaciously rather than being taken up with agitated thoughts and worries. At the same time we experience a sense of physical calmness in our bodies even if we are outwardly busy.

This kind of quietness can be seen as the opposite of anxiousness and overstimulation. We can't be anxious and quiet at the same time! Many of us have become so preoccupied with the demands and worries of our lives, or so addicted to stimulation, that our nervous system is in a near-constant state of anxious overwhelm. We've almost completely lost touch with what it means to be quiet in ourselves. Stress, tension and over-arousal have become the constant background to our existence.

Now and again people come for Alexander lessons having been encouraged to do so by friends or relations who are finding their stressful, tense state exasperating to live with. 'I can't understand it', the person says. 'I'm not stressed. I'm just busy. I don't feel tense at all.' But then after a few sessions, as their system starts to unwind, there's a sudden 'aha' moment. 'Ahhhh . . . now I see.' You can almost hear their loved ones sighing with them in relief.

When someone helps us experience this inner quietness, perhaps for the first time in many years, there's often a deep sense of recognition. Even if we can't remember having experienced it before, we instinctively know what it is and that it's right and good for us—just as we know that the sunlight filtering through the leaves of a forest, or the sound of waves quietly breaking on a beach, or relaxing into the embrace of a loved one is right and good for us. Perhaps it's reminiscent of the quietness we knew in the earliest days of our lives—or even before we were born—before we were caught up with worries, goals, hopes, expectations and fears and could just *be*, resting in the experience of each moment.

Presence

To become present is quite literally to 'come to our senses'. Think about being lost in a daydream—perhaps remembering something nice that happened yesterday or something tomorrow that you're looking forward to or worried about, so that your attention is completely taken up by the images in your head. You're conscious, but you're not really *here*. Lost in your inner world you've tuned out of your sensory experience in favour of the more abstract world of thought and imagination. If you were having an intimate conversation with a friend and they went off into such a daydream, you would probably experience it as a bit of an abandonment. There would be a sudden vacancy. 'Hey, where did you go?' you might say. Suddenly you're alone, even though the person is right in front of you.

Being taken up with our inner world—whether in a relaxed state of daydreaming or in a more focused state of thought or contemplation—is perfectly alright, of course. It's a necessary part of being human. But when tuning out of our senses becomes excessive and habitual it comes with a cost: we lose contact with the world as it actually is, with ourselves as *we* actually are, with other people, and with the lived experience of our life which is only ever happening now, in the present. At the same time we disconnect ourselves from the rich sensory data about ourselves and our relationship with the world around us that our system relies on to organise dynamic stabilisation, balance and support.

When we're not present we also lose much of our capacity to *choose*. We're on autopilot, leaving everything to habit. For many of us, those habits won't be ones that promote ease in ourselves and skilfulness in what we do.

All this is a shame because to be present is really a very simple thing—nothing more than deciding to be gently in touch with ourselves and the world around us through our eyes, touch and hearing, and through our proprioceptive senses that tell us how we are stabilising, balancing, feeling and moving from moment to moment. Being present like this we experience ourselves vibrantly, as palpable beings, in a real space, in relationship with tangible objects. We're in *this* body, in *these* surroundings, with *these* things, in *this* moment, *now*.

Openness

Presence is an essential quality of ease but it's not necessarily enough on its own. If you were caught in an earthquake or a fire, you might feel very intensely 'here' and in the moment, but that presence would quite likely not be accompanied by a state of ease and quietness!

When we're at ease, not only are we present but our field of attention is open and receptive, taking in what is happening inside and around us without unnecessary concentration and intentness. Our visual field in particular is mobile and free rather than fixed and staring, and our attention is free to move appropriately and easily from one sensory channel to another, shifting from sight to hearing to touch, to our sense of ourselves, our bodies, our movements and the surface of our skin. Our mental world of thoughts and feelings can take its natural place in this overall awareness without compromising our flexible, open connection with ourselves and the world around us.

When our attention is soft and open like this it's easier to be aware of more than one thing at a time. Sitting at our computer we may be aware of the words on the screen, our thoughts about them, the people passing by, the wind, the birds outside, the subtle movements of our body as it balances and finds support, and the feeling of the ground beneath our feet.

We've seen that whenever we narrow our field of attention by concentrating—whether voluntarily or spontaneously as a result of fear and anxiety—our musculature braces and tightens. This tightening is particularly noticeable in our eyes and head–neck joint, interfering with our ability to look freely, interestedly and openly around us. Our breath becomes tighter and shallower and our head freezes and fixes on our shoulders. When we look around us we may do so as if we were looking through a telescope, moving our narrowed field of vision rigidly from point to point. If our visual field of attention softens and broadens, on the other hand, our musculature softens too. Our eyes, head–neck joint and breathing spontaneously free up allowing us to take in more with each glance, while our head turns freely and easily in response to our interest.

Freedom

When we're in a state of ease, our musculature is unbraced, so we experience all the joints of our articulated structure as being free and available to move. Even if we're not actually moving right now, we have an intuitive sense that it would be easy and comfortable to go into movement at a moment's notice.

Free Breath

When our structure is in a free, unbraced state, our breath also moves freely without any sense of tightness and strain. Generally, we can leave it alone to spontaneously follow its own rhythm. But if we *do* need to voluntarily take a breath—for singing or swimming or some other reason—we experience that as free and easy too, with no undue sense of resistance or effort.

Because many of the muscles that play a role in breathing also help support and stabilise our structure, tightness and bracing anywhere in our body tends to be reflected by a degree of tightness and bracing in our breath too. When we come into a state of quiet, dynamic openness, on the other hand, our diaphragm and rib cage are free to move. Our belly muscles are free and unbraced leaving the diaphragm free to ascend and descend with each in-breath and out-breath, which we experience mostly second-hand through the delicate in-and-out movements of the belly that accompany it. Meanwhile, our ribcage is free to move delicately and easily too in the gentle bucket handle movement, which we experience as a delicate sideways expansion and contraction from the armpits to the bottom of the ribcage without any sense of tightness or strain.

All these subtle movements of the belly and ribs are experienced as light, free, integrated and unforced. They feel *good*. We may experience a pleasant sense of physical openness in our torso, across our ribcage and in the sensitive area around our belly and heart. At the same time we may notice that our voice becomes richer, deeper and stronger, and that the range of volume, pitch and tone available to us increases.

This openness and freedom in our belly, chest and voice can be quite lovely, but may also feel emotionally vulnerable to begin with. In time, though, vulnerability transforms into a new-found inner confidence and strength. Our increased physical openness may be mirrored in a feeling of being more emotionally open and available to others who may experience us as more expressive, open and engaging. We may laugh more often, and when we do, that laughter tends to be more uninhibited—and when we're sad it's easier to let go and sob if we need to.

Centredness

The four qualities I've described so far are found whenever our system is in a state of ease—whether we're upright and supported by our musculature or lying down with our muscles relaxed, supported entirely by the ground. The last three, though, are present only when we're upright, because they're a byproduct of being in a dynamic, responsive relationship with gravity.

The first of these is centredness. We've seen that to be in

a free and easy upright state, we need to be centred with our weight placed close to the middle of our base of support to avoid spontaneous protective bracing of our feet, legs and breath. Our weight doesn't need to be placed in the *exact* centre, though. In fact, if we tried to keep ourselves in such a precise position we would brace and freeze in the attempt. Rather, there's a comfortable, flexible *zone* around the middle of our base of support within which our system can spontaneously move and adjust to keep us balanced without overloading our muscles or triggering a protective bracing response.

There's a simple way to find this central zone. If you delicately shift your weight around over your base of support you'll find there's a small area within which your musculature spontaneously frees up a little. If you're standing, for example, you can sway around very slightly from your ankles and you'll find a place where there's a small release of tension in your feet, ankles, legs and breath.

If you're not used to this it can feel a little unnerving and insecure to begin with. Surely we need to make more effort than this to stay upright!

But actually, it's *more* secure. Being centred you have further to go before losing your balance, and your balance responses are freer to make delicate spontaneous adjustments to keep you in equilibrium. In time, you'll find a different, more flexible, alive and responsive sense of security in this more centred place.

Dynamic Stabilisation

When we're upright and at ease our system stabilises us dynamically. We experience this in the subtle, spontaneous adjustments of muscle tone that are constantly going on throughout us, matching the forces impinging on us as we breathe, balance and move about. This constant subtle movement creates a sense of delicate *aliveness* in the body.

Do you know the lithe, fluid quality that many animals tend to exhibit as a matter of course? If you gently put a hand on a horse, or a cat or dog, there's usually an acute sense of being in contact with a vibrant, living being as their system responds sensitively to you, to gravity and to the world around them. This is what *we're* like when our system is balancing and stabilising us in a dynamic way. It feels quite different to the rigid, stiff, immobile quality you experience if you put a hand on many adult humans who have got into the habit of supporting themselves through bracing and rigidity.

These subtle, ongoing spontaneous movements of dynamic stabilisation have a living, *unpredictable* quality. They always seem fresh and new because they're not being done deliberately by us as an act of will. They happen on their own as our body responds to the demands of each moment, independently of anything that we, as a separate, observing I, may be wanting or expecting of them.

Grounded Support

When we're upright and in a state of ease, our relationship with gravity seems relaxed, effortless and easy too. We're not needing to brace and hold ourselves to remain upright. Instead we experience a comfortable, lively connection with the ground allied with a sense of rising lightness and support.

Grounded support activates from our contact with the surface beneath us—from our feet when we're standing, our sitting bones when we're sitting, our hands and feet when we're on all fours, or from whatever other parts of us are bearing our weight at any given moment. As we've seen, when we're upright and at ease, a chain of dynamic support can travel from these points of contact up through each load-bearing joint of our structure, while the absence of bracing and unnecessary muscular contraction allows our spine to spontaneously assume its full, unforced length and our head to balance freely and easily on top.

There's no need to *do* anything to bring all this about. Think how absurd it would be for cats or dogs to go around thinking about the right way to curve their spines or hold their heads! They allow their system to organise it for them while they get on with investigating, hunting, eating or whatever else they're up to. So long as we create the right conditions and aren't consciously or unconsciously interfering with it, we can trust our system to organise dynamic, grounded support for us, too.

When we're standing, grounded support begins with our feet resting freely and easily on the floor, our weight distributed over a triangle made of the ball of the foot, the heel and the foot's outside edge. Our nervous system gets important sensory information from this free, flexible contact, helping it to accurately gauge whether we're in balance and how our weight is placed from moment to moment. Dynamic support can then activate from our feet, travelling up from joint to joint—through ankles, knees, hips, from vertebra to vertebra, right up to the head–neck joint at the top.

Similar principles operate whenever we're at ease and in an upright, active relationship with gravity. If we're sitting in a chair, for example, the main point of physical and sensory contact with the surface beneath us is the two rocker-shaped 'sitting bones' on each side of our pelvis. Grounded support can activate from that contact, through the hip joints, travelling up the spine to our head. It's similar if we're on all fours. Effectively we now have *four* feet. If we allow it, dynamic support can travel up from each one—from our knees to our hip joints and from our hands through our wrists, elbows and shoulder joints. Muscles spontaneously activate to dynamically support the shoulder girdle and spine, delicately suspending our torso between our front legs, just as happens for other four-legged animals.

Some of us tend to have a rather collapsed, heavy relationship with the ground. This may be related to a disconnection from our sense of ourselves and our surroundings, which starves our system of the sensory information it needs to organise in a dynamic way. Often there's an emotional component, too. If we tend to feel low and deflated, or that we're not worth very much, this may be reflected in a low-energy, collapsed, unsupported state. Or we may manifest physically the way we feel emotionally by unconsciously *pulling* our head and torso downwards, leading to a tight, braced hunch.

For others, a lack of grounded support may come from the opposite impulse—from a subtle sense of pulling *up*, off and *away* from the ground. This may be with our feet—our arches, toes or heels curling and pulling upwards—or we may pull up and away from the Earth with our coccyx or breastbone. This pattern is often present when things have happened that made the world feel unsafe—particularly if they happened when we were very young.* It may be accompanied by a feeling of being

---

* See Chapter Thirty-One for more about this.

somewhat detached—not just from the ground but from life itself. We may subconsciously feel that we're not welcome, or that we don't quite belong or have a right to be here. It may feel safer or less painful to not quite land and be a fully engaged participant in life on Earth.

If we aren't used to accessing grounded support, learning to do so can be like entering a new world. We may experience the ascending chain of support almost as if it were some subtle energy flowing up through us from the floor to our head. The responsive, sensitive, weight-bearing contact with the ground tends to make us feel connected, present and fully here, while the rising dynamic support makes us feel simultaneously light, flexible, strong and free. We may even literally grow a little taller as our spine decompresses into its full length.

Some people may find this makes them feel uncomfortably conspicuous to begin with. It may feel as if allowing themselves to be their full height will make others think they're arrogant and 'too big for their boots'. But as we get accustomed to it we see that what we're experiencing is simply a healthy sense of self-esteem and confidence. We realise that, like any other creature, we have the right to unashamedly take up space and allow ourselves to comfortably adopt our full size.

Chapter Fifteen
Four Characteristics of Skilful Action

Let it be whatever you want, but at least let it be unified.
—HORACE, 'The Art of Poetry'

In the last couple of chapters I've encouraged you to imagine yourself in a state of ease and to think about what that state would be like and what its qualities would be. To keep things simple, I suggested that you assumed you weren't doing much in this state—just sitting or standing quietly, in neutral. This is fine as far as it goes, but of course sooner or later you *would* want to do things, and hopefully you'd be taking that state of ease with you into the activity so that your movements would also exhibit the lovely free, open quality that comes when our system is in a state of freedom and dynamic stabilisation and support.

So let's imagine once again that you're in a quiet, present state of ease, but this time while involved in some skilful pastime: running lightly and easily through a park, perhaps, or playing a musical instrument with a little flair and sensitivity, or just having a walk in the woods, moving easily along, delicately in tune with your body and the sights and sounds all around you. Or perhaps in your imagination you're interacting skilfully with another person, dancing harmoniously with each other, or playing duets at the piano, or being intimate together with a sense of genuine contact, connection and playfulness.

For a start, all the qualities of ease would still be there. There would still be quietness, presence, openness, freedom, centredness, dynamic stabilisation and grounded support manifesting from moment to moment. But for these qualities to *continue* into the activity, your movements would need to be coordinated in ways that wouldn't cause your musculature to spontaneously brace and tighten. Skilful movement has several characteristics that help prevent this from happening. In particular:

1. **Integration.** When we move skilfully, many joints and muscles work elegantly and sensitively together, co-ordinating all-of-a-piece to distribute muscular effort throughout the body.

2. **Centredness.** Skilful movements are coordinated in ways that keep us centred as we go, keeping our weight close to the middle of our base of support no matter how complex the activity we're engaged in.

3. **Economy.** Skilful movement avoids unnecessary muscular effort, using innate movement patterns and gravity and momentum to help if needed.

4. **Flow.** When we're moving skilfully our movements flow freely from one to another without holding and bracing in between. To facilitate this we may find ourselves pre-emptively shifting our weight or placing our limbs for support so as to enable ease in the more goal-directed movements that follow.

Let's look at each of these in turn.

Integration

To move easily and skilfully, many muscles and joints need to work together, giving our actions a light, sensitive, fluid, joined-up quality. If we reach out for something we may do so with a single economical unfolding of our whole arm—the shoulder joint, shoulder blade, elbow, wrist, fingers and rotation of the forearm all working together, accompanied, perhaps, by a very slight leaning back from the ankles, or a subtle rotation of the spine and pelvis, to counterbalance the weight of our extending arm, keeping us centred as we go. Everything works together. Similarly, if we were to turn to look behind us, our head, spine, pelvis and legs would all move together creating one integrated coordination. If we wanted to roll over in bed, or move from lying on our side onto all fours, the work would be shared between our torso, head, arms and legs, all skilfully coordinating, pushing, yielding and shifting as needed, distributing effort to create a single easy, fluid action. And if we want to move into standing, or down into sitting or a crouch, our ankle joints, knees and hip joints would fold or unfold together in a single light, harmonious, concertina-like movement.

Many of us, though, have got into the habit of moving in unintegrated, fragmented ways. We may brace some joints rigidly as we move—holding on in some places to support movement in others. If we reach out for something with an arm, we might fix our elbow so that the movement occurs entirely at the shoulder joint, giving it a rather club-like quality. Turning to look behind us, we might turn only our head and shoulders while bracing our torso, pelvis and legs, resulting in a rather stiff movement with a limited range. Getting up from the ground onto all fours or rolling over in bed, we may forcefully twist our torso around without offering sufficient help from a pushing or supporting arm or leg. And when we stand up or sit down in a chair, the movement may be broken up into chunks rather than flowing together as one.

Do you remember we saw earlier that when our muscles are put under significant load it evokes a spontaneous bracing response? One consequence of fragmented movement patterns is that they can easily put us into positions in which our muscles brace through becoming overloaded *by our own body weight*. Our body parts are heavy, and when we move or hold ourselves in ways that require a few muscles to support a substantial part of that weight it can generate forces that are sufficient to trigger this response.

Say I'm lying on my back, and I decide to sit up by hauling my head and torso straight up off the ground. Muscles in my torso, and particularly my belly, will suddenly have to support the entire weight of my torso and head, causing them to brace fiercely. Try it now. It's easy to notice. Or say I'm lying on my back and I lift an outstretched arm or leg straight off the floor from the shoulder or hip joint. The weight will overload my muscles causing some bracing in the limb itself and in my torso and breath. There are all sorts ways—some very obvious, others rather subtle—in which unintegrated, fragmented movement patterns can trigger unintended bracing like this.

When we move skilfully we avoid movements that overload our muscles, choosing ways of coordinating ourselves that achieve our aims while distributing muscular effort widely instead, creating a sense of ease and lightness because no one part of us is being overworked. We fold and unfold, reaching and retracting, pushing and yielding sensitively with our limbs where it's needed to support the weight of other body parts—spiralling, gesturing, balancing and breathing all-of-a-piece. We'll explore how we can go about finding ways of moving like this in Part Four of the book.

Centredness

We've already seen that centredness is an essential quality of ease, so to act skilfully the movements of our limbs, torso and head need to be coordinated in ways that *keep* us centred, so that our weight stays close to the middle of our base of support as we go.

If I want to reach out my hand for something, for example, some kind of compensatory movement will be needed to counterbalance the weight of my outstretched arm—perhaps a slight shift backwards from my ankles or a complementary movement backwards with the other arm. Or think about getting up from a chair. Often as people stand up they begin pushing to straighten their legs very early in the movement while their weight is still some way behind their feet. This puts significant loads onto their ankles, knees and hip joints causing their muscles to brace fiercely to prevent them falling backwards. Their legs tighten, their lower back arches and their head is pulled back and down. Any chance of getting out of the chair with freedom and ease is lost.

Or think about taking a step forwards. We need to become briefly one-legged as we lift the stepping leg off the ground. Often people lift their leg to take the step before their weight has shifted onto the other one, causing muscles in their legs, pelvis and belly to brace to stabilise the suddenly unbalanced load. To take a step while allowing dynamic stabilisation and grounded support to continue through the movement, our weight needs to shift onto the supporting leg, centring us there while unloading the other one so we can take the step freely and easily.*

Considering all the complex ways our body parts can move in relation to each other, you might imagine that staying centred in activity must be very difficult, but it's simpler than you might think. Like all animals we seem to have an innate understanding of gravity and movement. We know intuitively whether a particular movement would take us out of balance and cause us to fall. It only takes a little bit of extra sensitivity and refinement to make sure that our weight stays close to the centre of our base of support rather than shifting uncomfortably near to the edge as we move. Later on, in Chapter Twenty-Four, I'll tell you about a simple way to begin to access this sensitivity and refinement for yourself.

Economy

Skilful movement is economical and doesn't waste energy. When we're moving skilfully we don't thud heavily as we walk, or push forcefully with our legs to haul ourselves up the stairs. We don't effortfully grip, push or pull things if we don't need to—we use no more force than is necessary. If we're playing the violin we don't grip the neck fiercely, if we're playing the piano we don't prod our fingers heavily into the keybed, and if we're carrying something heavy we keep it close to our body rather than making our muscles work unnecessarily hard by holding it at a distance. We avoid excess effort wherever we can so that our movements are light, easy and free.

---

* When we're walking at speed, our momentum carries us forwards so our weight doesn't need to shift nearly so much with each step.

Innate Movement Patterns

I mentioned in Chapter Nine that certain ways of coordinating our movements are hardwired into us. These innate movement patterns evolved to make the most efficient use of our muscles and structure, motor programmes and muscle synergies combining to make movement seem effortless if we can only get out of their way and allow them to operate freely. I can think of moving my hand towards something and back again, for example, and allow the complex unfolding movement of my arm to elegantly self-organise in response to this simple wish. Similarly, if I'm wanting to look behind me I can turn my head and allow my torso, pelvis and legs to follow its movement freely. Or if I want to reach down to pick something up from the floor, I can let my ankle, knee and hip joints fold in a single, integrated concertina-like action. It's interesting to experiment and discover other ways in which our body will respond in a complex, integrated manner to our simpler intentions.

I also mentioned central pattern generators which can automatically organise some common repetitive movement patterns such as walking and running. These also evolved to make economical use of our anatomy and require a minimum of mental and physical effort. When we walk or run—or even if we're just taking a single step—we can allow the stepping movements, and the subtle rotational movements of the pelvis and torso that go with them, to unfold freely on their own. If we can get out of their way it can feel almost as if we're being *carried* by our legs rather than effortfully moving them to get about. Likewise, if we're standing and want to turn around, we can allow our system to place our feet and move our legs as needed to keep up with the turn. Given a chance our body will sort out the necessary stepping and shifting movements spontaneously. It's surprising how subtle and effective these spontaneous adjustments can be if the body is really left to its own devices.

Gravity and Momentum

Sometimes we can take advantage of gravity and momentum to facilitate economical movement. When we're walking, for example, we can let our arms swing freely, allowing gravity to swing them down and momentum to swing them back up again like pendulums. Our muscles don't have to do very much to keep them going.

We can also sometimes use our body weight to help us move. This can be particularly helpful in recumbent movements. Say we're lying flat on our back. It can be a little awkward to roll over onto our side just by twisting our head and torso, even if we give them some help by pushing with an arm or leg. But if we bring our legs up we can then tip them to one side and their weight will help to carry us over. We can also use the weight of our arms to help with lots of different rolling movements by moving the opposite arm across our body in the direction we want to roll, or by extending the arm on the side we're rolling onto and lifting it a little, keeping it off the ground as we go.

Momentum can be useful too, enabling us to initiate movements with a burst of energy before allowing them to continue on their own, giving us time to recover and reset so that our attention and energy can be gathered at the end of the movement where we need the most precision and control. If I want to spin around on the spot, for example, I can spread my arms and swing them to get me going, allowing their momentum to carry me round before applying effort again when I want to bring myself to a stop. Similarly, a skilled gymnast can learn to trust momentum to carry them through the air so they can release and reset their musculature as they go, giving them a chance to prepare a dynamic, attuned landing.

We can even use momentum to our advantage in a simple movement like standing up from a chair. If we come forwards swiftly from our hip joints, the forward momentum of our head and torso will enable us to begin straightening our legs without bracing or falling backwards, even before our weight is fully over our feet. By the time it arrives there, we're already upright.

Flow

Skilful activity *flows*. We move freely and easily from movement to movement without bracing in between, and when we come to rest we're already at ease, ready to move freely off again as and when we need to.

Preparative Movements

Flow often depends on how we sequence smaller movements to achieve our larger goals. Roughly speaking, we can divide our movements into two categories. Some are aimed directly at achieving our aims—reaching for the plates when washing up, pressing the keys on the piano, taking steps as we walk across the room. I call these '**goal-directed movements**'. They're the ones we tend to be most concerned with and aware of. But there's another class of movements, which I call **preparative movements**, which involve placing our limbs or shifting our weight as needed to facilitate ease in the more obviously goal-directed ones that follow. We've already come across several examples of situations where we need to make preparative movements like this. If I'm standing and want to take a step, for example, I'll need to shift my weight onto the supporting leg first so that I don't tighten up or fall over as I lift the other one off the ground; if I want to stand up from a chair I'll first need to lean forwards to shift my weight over my feet or I'll fall backwards as I try to straighten my legs; if I'm lying on my back and want to use the weight of my legs to help me roll onto my side, I'll need to bend and raise them before I can let them fall sideways to carry me over; if I want to pick something up from a table, I might step towards it with one foot, centring myself there as I reach out with my arms so that I don't need to stretch too far; and if I'm lying on my side and want to come up onto all fours, I may place my hands or legs sensitively on the ground first so that I can use them to help me roll over, pushing and yielding as needed to share the load, rather than relying on forcefully bending, lifting and twisting my torso and head.

We saw earlier that many of us have a strong tendency to endgain, hurrying towards our goals without paying enough attention to the process we are using to get there. One common way that endgaining manifests is by us rushing though the preparative shifting and placing movements that are needed to facilitate ease as we proceed towards our goal—or even omitting them altogether. If we're going to stay free and unbraced in activity, our preparative movements are as important as the goal-directed ones that come after them. There needs to be a clarity about the necessary order of things as we sensitively and accurately move to centre ourselves and place our limbs in support of the more goal-directed movements that follow. When we're moving really freely, it can even come to seem, paradoxically, as if these preparative movements are the most important ones of all—as if what we're *actually* up to is moving from one well-supported, well-centred, well-prepared place to another via our goal-directed movements, rather than the other way round, resulting in an unfolding sense of ease, lightness and flow in whatever we do.

Chapter Sixteen
Paradise Lost

So far in this book I've been suggesting that our body and nervous system evolved to spontaneously organise ease and dynamic support for us as we go about our lives. Soon we'll be exploring steps you can take to rediscover that ease for yourself. But first I want to give a little more space to understanding how things tend to go wrong for so many of us, preventing our system from organising freely and easily as it should.

We've already touched on various things that can get in the way of ease, such as fear and anxiety, endgaining, sensory disengagement, concentration, unhelpful movement patterns and unnecessary voluntary interference with stabilisation, support and breathing. In addition, our ability to manifest ease may be compromised due to the effects of past traumatic experiences and suppressed or repressed emotions. We're affected by these and other factors to varying degrees according to our life experience, environment, personality and genetic makeup. Some of us get off relatively lightly. The patterns of interference we've picked up aren't too deep and are relatively easy to unpick. Others may have developed deeper and more complex patterns of intertwined muscular and emotional holding which may take longer to resolve. We can all benefit, though, from understanding the origins and causes of unhelpful habits and patterns we've got ourselves into.

More About Anxiety

Modern people live under very different social and economic circumstances to those we evolved to deal with. Rather than spending our lives in small, cohesive tribes where everyone depends on everyone else, we must navigate a complex, fragmented social world that's in constant flux. Partly because of this, many of us—even those who are generally happy or successful—have come to feel somewhat *unsafe* in a deep part of ourselves. There's a sense of insecurity about our lives, finances and relationships. This may begin with the transition away from the family when we start school, in our teenage years, or as we start to face the uncertainty of adult life. And unfortunately, some are born into such difficult, deprived or abusive situations that they may never have had the experience of feeling truly safe and secure at all.

As well as this, we tend to be exposed to constant comparison to others on the grounds of class, race, competence, attractiveness and wealth—not just by those around us but through the media, which bombards us with unrealistic ideals of beauty and attainment. Many of us are left with the uneasy feeling that we are fundamentally not OK—that we're not enough or loveable as we are. All of this can engender an ongoing sense of anxiety.

This kind of anxiety is different from fear. Fear is a response to immediate danger—the leopard passing in the jungle or the sound of a window breaking downstairs in your house at night. It's a response to direct physical threats which are happening *now*. Anxiety is more about what we imagine may happen to us in the future. Perhaps we imagine losing status, money, security or the love and respect of others. Though these things may not be happening at the moment, our body responds to these imagined threats as if they were immediate physical dangers, arousing us to prepare for an immediate physical response. But unlike with a passing leopard or the noise in the night, these threats often don't pass quickly and there's usually nothing about them that can be solved through immediate physical action anyway. We wake each morning faced with the same worrying possibilities.

Learned Fear Responses

The kind of anxieties I've been describing above come from our high-level mental world of thoughts and images. We imagine worrying scenarios, and our bodies respond as if the imagined danger were a real, physical threat. But there's another way our primitive defensive responses can get activated, even though there's no danger present in the here and now, which originates from negative past experiences retained by *low*-level parts of the brain.

When we have a very unpleasant or frightening experience, our limbic brain stores it up. If we come across another situation that seems similar, it instantly triggers a defensive response causing our body to prepare to fight, flee, freeze or flop before our higher-level conscious brain even recognises what's happening. This is called a **learned fear response**. While these serve important purposes for survival, they can also cause our system to respond to non-life-threatening situations in unhelpful ways. Suppose we've been badly hurt in our relationships. We may feel anxious if we find ourselves getting into a new one that looks like it's becoming serious—or even if we just meet someone who reminds us of a person who hurt us. We may suddenly pull away, shut down or lash out angrily, much to the other person's mystification and dismay.

Learned fear responses often play a role in difficulties in performance situations such as public speaking, sports or music and other artistic endeavours. But anything that reminds our brain of a difficult or unpleasant past experience may cause our primitive defensive responses to activate. Say that when we were at school we were humiliated for making mistakes or failing to come up to other people's expectations. Any learning situations that we encounter later on may trigger fear, anxiety and shame making the task of learning much harder, or limiting us by causing us to avoid learning new things altogether. Even apparently light-hearted disparagement of a young person's efforts can have these kinds of long-term consequences.

Anxiety and Busyness

Some people are anxious a lot of the time and are well aware of it. They know they are often worried and on edge. This persistent over-arousal may leave them jittery and restless, or it can have a fixed, frozen quality as their system remains activated for self-defensive action that never comes. But anxiety can also manifest in a less obvious way, in the form of a driven, obsessive *busyness* which the person may even view as a positive thing.

Of course, there's nothing inherently wrong with being busy and productive, but sometimes busyness is excessive, driven by hidden fears and anxieties rather than real needs. Perhaps we unconsciously believe that we must be constantly, frenetically busy to survive financially even when this isn't the case. Or we may fear that recognition, love and respect from others depend on us doing and achieving certain things, leaving us in a state of continuous struggle to meet these real or imagined criteria for acceptance. Although it may be less obvious than overt anxiety, this kind of busy, driven anxiousness is just as unhelpful, preventing dynamic muscular organisation from activating and getting in the way of the quiet calmness and presence needed to be in the world with skilfulness and ease.

Problems with Presence and Attention

We've seen that the dynamic stabilisation that underpins ease and skilfulness is dependent on our senses. Our system needs sensory information to ascertain our orientation and alignment in space, to accurately gauge the position and movement of our body parts, and to sense the amount of muscular tension being applied from moment to moment. If it doesn't get enough of that information to enable it to organise dynamically it has no option but to resort to simpler, braced stabilisation strategies instead.

We also saw that acquiring this sensory information is facilitated by us being open and present to ourselves and our surroundings. But many people find this difficult. Habitual rushing and impatience prevent us from being present to where we are and what we're doing. Habitual concentration narrows our field of awareness. And boredom can cause us to tune out of our experience of the present moment as we seek stimulation in our inner world.

Impatience and Rushing

Rushing is not the same thing as acting swiftly. We can do things quickly and efficiently without being in a rush. Rushing, on the other hand, is a form of endgaining that happens when we get mentally ahead of ourselves, straining to get onto the next step rather than being with the step we're on and with what needs doing right now, at *this* moment.

Rushing is often a side effect of boredom. If we're not interested and engaged in a task, we're more likely to rush to get it over quickly, making a hurried and slapdash job of it. Often we learn to rush at school if we're continually made to do things which feel nonsensical, irrelevant or uncomfortable. We might tend to try and get these unpleasant tasks over with as quickly as possible. In time, disengagement and rushing may become such ingrained habits that we bring them even to tasks we care about.

Tuning Out

Many of us spend too much of our lives doing things that aren't very stimulating in surroundings that are uninspiring or unpleasant. Think of those demoralising jobs where we turn up day after day at an impersonal office or factory to do tasks we don't enjoy and that have no inherent meaning for us. Or perhaps we're in an unhappy relationship, or having to deal with other demands which we find challenging and difficult. Mentally, physically and spiritually, we're uncomfortable. The day becomes a thing to get through with gritted teeth.

One way to make such situations more tolerable is to escape into our heads. We tune out of our experience of the present and think about other things. We plan for the future or worry about the news. We remember things that happened in the past or ruminate on our current problems and difficulties.

This disengagement from our senses often starts early. Children are born with the innate curiosity, interest and capacity to enjoy life but are often pushed too early into commodified education that doesn't consider them as individuals or engage their interest. This may be exacerbated by their being expected to sit still and focus for long periods on tasks they experience as irrelevant and dull before their minds and bodies have developed sufficiently to enable them to comfortably do so. The boredom and physical discomfort that results may be a strong incentive for them to tune out of their bodily awareness and spend the time lost in their thoughts instead. This can be a difficult habit to break later on.

Concentration

I'm sure you've got the idea by now that although there are some situations when concentration is helpful and appropriate, most of the time it does more harm than good. In spite of this, it's often portrayed as a positive thing associated with the ability to focus on a task in a disciplined way. Of course, we *do* all need to be able to focus and not be waylaid by every passing whim or distraction. But there's a big difference between gently but persistently choosing to stay on task and concentrating in the sense of rigidly narrowing and fixing our attention. Many of us have developed such a strong habit of doing this that it happens whenever we engage in any task that involves the slightest level of manual or intellectual skill. At worst, it can become our default way of being in the world which is activated almost continuously no matter what we are doing.

We've seem that concentration can be a particular problem in skilled, complex activities like sport or the arts where it gets in the way of the open, flexible, inclusive awareness that's necessary to perform well. The irony in this is that many of us concentrate because of a deep, subconscious assumption that it helps us to achieve more and be better at things. This attitude is often taught to us when we're young. At school we may have been told to concentrate on our lessons and may have come to sincerely believe that it helps us. This is reinforced throughout our lives. We're told that we should 'try hard' and 'make an effort' if we're to succeed in life. It's easy to interpret this as an instruction to concentrate—even though the habit of inappropriate concentration actually makes whatever we're doing considerably more difficult and less enjoyable.

Voluntary Interference

The factors we've looked at so far affect our systems for stabilisation and support indirectly. But people often interfere with these systems directly too, voluntarily holding themselves rigidly in their attempts to look better or to ameliorate everyday discomfort and pain. In time, this voluntary interference can become habitual so that it's continually being triggered outside of our conscious awareness.

Deliberate Interference

Many people develop the habit of deliberately bracing their posture in the belief it will help them to be more comfortable, look better or improve their health. We pick up all sorts of ideas about what 'good posture' is from well-meaning teachers, parents and the culture at large and believe we should be doing things to maintain it, such as pulling our shoulders back, tucking our tailbone in, 'sitting up straight' or whatever other ideas are fashionable at the moment. While it might superficially seem like common sense, this voluntary maintenance of posture is counterproductive.

Try it now. Sit up really straight, whatever you imagine that to involve. Can you see that while you may seem somewhat more upright, what you're actually doing is bracing yourself using muscles that are optimised for movement rather than support, tightening them against each other so that your structure becomes fixed and held? You may believe that you're improving your posture by doing this, but really you're making yourself rigid, interfering with the natural rhythm of breathing, and compromising your body's innate tendency to organise dynamic stabilisation and support. In the process, you're putting your muscles, joints and internal organs under a great deal of unnecessary stress and strain.

Subconscious Interference

Apart from consciously bracing and holding our posture according to ideas we've picked up from others, we may also voluntarily hold and brace ourselves in less explicitly thought-through ways. This may begin with being uncomfortable due to sitting or standing in one position for an unnaturally long time for work or leisure activities. Humans have a surprising ability to ignore their body's distress signals and stay on task for prolonged periods despite sometimes quite extreme physical discomfort. It's strange if you think about it. Other animals don't force themselves to stay in one position for hours on end. If they become uncomfortable they get up and move about, or lie down and have a rest. We humans, however, tend to keep going despite the discomfort. We 'push on through' rather than taking a break and giving our bodies a chance to recover. Instead of taking time out, we semi-consciously shift ourselves about, finding ways of holding ourselves that reduce our discomfort temporarily while allowing us to continue with whatever task we're compulsively pursuing.

Many people—particularly those who live very desk-bound lives—get into cycles of repetitive bracing and collapse throughout the day. They brace to hold themselves upright until, after a while, their muscles tire and they let go into a slump. Then they feel guilty and sit up straight again until they get tired and collapse once more, round and round throughout the day. Walk around an office at the end of the day and you'll find people braced or collapsed into the most extraordinarily contorted positions. Over time, these ways of holding ourselves can become embedded and habitual. Though we started doing them with at least some degree of background awareness, they end up becoming automatic, continuing even when they no longer offer even temporary relief from the discomfort we feel.

Emotional Suppression and Repression

When we're very young we're at the mercy of our emotions. If we're sad, we cry; if we're angry, we yell; if we're happy, we laugh. We depend completely on others to help calm and soothe us if we get upset, angry, frightened or overexcited. But as we get older we often need to be able to voluntarily put our moment-to-moment emotional responses aside for the good of the group or the task at hand. Voluntarily controlling our emotions like this is called **suppression,** and it's an essential adult skill. If, following an argument with our partner, we need to get in our car and drive somewhere, it's important to be able to park our feelings rather than express them freely by ranting and raving at other road users. For a sports team to play well, each member needs to be able to keep their individual excitement in check and work for the good of the team as a whole. And imagine the chaos that would ensue if a couple raising a baby gave free rein to every passing emotion like their child did!

We may also suppress our emotions for less healthy reasons. We might discover, for example, that it's safer to suppress our natural reactions to avoid the judgement of others. If crying or expressions of anger or sadness are seen as unacceptable manifestations of weakness or defiance by those around us, then expressing these emotions may make us vulnerable to shaming or some other form of unpleasantness, and so we may suppress them instead. Similarly, if we have an urge to laugh loudly or to spontaneously sing or dance but have experienced wounding barbs and put-downs when we've done so in the past, we may feel it's best to suppress the wish to do so.

Subtle or obvious disapproval of physical movement and self-expression is a significant force in many modern cultures, so apart from suppressing strong emotions like anger or sadness we may also get into the habit of suppressing more subtle impulses such as stretching, sighing, yawning, wriggling, groaning with frustration or laughing in a truly full and open-hearted way. This is a shame because these impulses arise for important reasons—to help prevent stronger feelings from building up, to re-organise muscle tone in our system and to encourage accumulated emotional and muscular tension to let go. Can you imagine a dog or a cat deciding not to have a good stretch or growl when they feel like it in case of what other animals might think? They're happy to be themselves and allow their body to move and express itself as it needs to. As much as possible it's best for us to do the same.

Suppression Versus Repression

Suppression is possible because much of our emotional expression takes place through our body. Whether we're crying with sadness or joy, trembling with rage, shaking with anger or fear, or laughing with happiness, the experience is always to some extent embodied and physical. This means we can often block an emotional response by blocking the movements or bodily responses accompanying it. If we're sad and don't want to cry, we may hold our shoulders firmly to prevent the rhythmic motions of sobbing, and force ourselves to 'hold back the tears'. If we're fearful we may try to keep a 'stiff upper lip' and hold on to our pelvis, legs and shoulders to prevent shaking and shuddering. We may tighten the muscles of our face to hold back the facial expressions that go along with sadness or shame and tighten our mouth and throat to prevent spontaneous vocalisation of alarm, sadness or distress.

Hopefully, when we suppress our emotional responses it's for a good reason and later, when we're in a situation where it's safe and appropriate, we'll allow ourselves to experience the feelings and let them go. Maybe we'll have a good cry, or rant to a friend and feel better. But it may not always be so simple. What if there's no safe place to let the feelings go? Perhaps no one in our lives would be willing to witness them with us. Or maybe what's happening is so serious, and the emotions are so big, that we subconsciously fear they'll overwhelm us or be unbearable to acknowledge and experience. Or maybe we've been conditioned to believe that certain emotions, feelings or desires are so inherently wrong and shameful that we not only can't bring ourselves to express them, but can't admit to ourselves that we have them at all.

In such cases, the emotions can become disowned and **repressed**. We may deny them even to ourselves so that they become unconscious, locked in our bodies and minds through muscular tension.[*] This not only interferes with our body's attempts to organise in an easy, dynamic way but also with our ability to express ourselves as open, sensitive beings, making certain forms of emotional experience difficult to access.

If we're holding repressed emotions in our body, a practice like the Alexander Technique can encourage the associated muscular bracing to release, allowing the feelings to finally be let go of. As part of this process, there can be a period during a course of lessons when a person feels unaccountably weepy, sad or angry as the emotions dissipate and resolve. There is more about this process later on in the book.[†]

---

[*] Wilhelm Reich called this chronic, emotionally-based muscular bracing 'armouring', because it makes our musculature rigid in an attempt to protect ourselves and others from our negative feelings.

[†] When people have had particularly difficult experiences in their past, they may need more specialised therapeutic help to enable them to let the very strong stored feelings resolve in a safe, contained way.

Chapter Seventeen
Unreliable Sensory Appreciation

You can't know a thing by an instrument that's wrong.
—F.M. ALEXANDER, Aphorisms

Bracing and excess muscular tension is a common thread that connects all the things we've identified so far that get in the way of our body's innate tendency to manifest ease. But, over time, chronic muscular bracing has other, more subtle effects. In particular, it can cause our proprioceptive senses to become unreliable, affecting the accuracy with which we perceive the alignment of our body segments, our relationship to gravity, and the muscular effort required to move and support ourselves. At the same time, chronic bracing can cause our internal mental picture of our structure, or '**body map**', to become inaccurate, which can have significant negative effects on how we move and function. F.M. Alexander called these various sensory mismatches and errors **unreliable sensory appreciation**.

Sense of Alignment, Balance and Effort

Generally, the way someone habitually sits or stands feels upright and aligned to them even if it is not. Perhaps we tend to stand leaning forwards, or with just our hips pushed forwards making us slightly banana-shaped, or we habitually sit with an exaggerated concave curve in our lower back. If so, there's a good chance we'll be unaware of it. People often come for Alexander lessons with habits like this. If the teacher takes a photo to show them how they're holding themselves, the person will frequently be astonished at the mismatch between how they feel and how they actually are. Not only that, but if the teacher gently helps them shift towards a more aligned, balanced state, the person may, to begin with, feel crooked, out of balance and wrong!

It's also common that when we spend a lot of time with our musculature braced for support, the excess effort comes to feel not only normal but *necessary*. This can present a barrier to improving things because it may feel as if stopping all that bracing would cause us to collapse and fall down. Similarly, when our musculature is chronically braced and contracted we tend to use a lot more effort to move than we need to. Over time we can become so habituated to this unnecessary force in our movements that it may feel not only strange but *impossible* to move without it.

Some people know all too well that their muscles are uncomfortably tense and held a lot of the time. But it's also possible to lose touch with these sensations of tension, becoming so used to them that they no longer feel remarkable. The excess tension comes to feel normal, leaving the person unaware that their muscles are in a state of constant over-contraction and strain.

The Body Map and Movement

Another side effect of chronic muscular bracing is that it tends to affect our mental picture of how our body is put together. Alexander teachers call this mental picture our 'body map'. Many of our muscles cross multiple joints, particularly in our torso and neck where there are many small bones in close proximity. When these muscles brace they can lock groups of joints together, effectively making them into rigid blocks so that some of the joints within the block are fixed and unavailable for movement.

Say you were sitting down and wanted to lean forwards to reach for something, but your hip joints were braced, locking your pelvis and legs rigidly together. You'd have to make the leaning movement from your lumbar spine instead, even though your hip joints are better designed and positioned for the job. Or if the head–neck joint between your spine and skull was braced, you may have to shift nodding and head-turning movements to lower down your neck or even to your torso. Similarly, braced muscles in your back, arms and shoulder blades may substantially immobilise your shoulder girdle, leaving you unaware of its capacity for sensitive movement. This can end up with your arms hanging as if your shoulders were a dead mass rather than the sensitive, pliable partners for your arms that they evolved to be.

Bracing our structure into chunks like this not only limits our capacity for ease and fluidity but also undermines our *perception* of our body and how it can move. We begin to picture it as if the limited, constrained experience of movement we're having reflects its true nature. We come to see our shoulder girdle as a blocky, amorphous, rigid part of our torso rather than as the potentially flexible, sensitive structure it actually is. We start to believe that our head–neck joint really is somewhere at the base of our neck and that our hip joints really are located somewhere at the top of our pelvis—to the extent that if someone were to ask us to show them where these key joints are located we'd point to the wrong place!

Even if the bracing that caused our body map to become inaccurate is removed we may still move according to that faulty map, because it's become lodged in our brain where it's gained a life of its own independent of our body. Later on I'll tell you about a practice called **body mapping** that can help you to gently correct your body map so that it more accurately reflects your true structure, becoming an accurate guide for the movements you make and the things you want to do.

Chapter Eighteen
The Tangled Thread

Even someone who's managed to retain a degree of ease and skilfulness as they've gone through life can experience moments when anxiousness, misdirected attention, insecure balance or voluntary bracing interfere with their body's capacity for dynamic ease, stabilisation and support. They can lose their equilibrium and become momentarily rather tense and awkward. But for them, getting back on track tends to be fairly straightforward. They notice they're getting overanxious and intent and take a moment to calm down and let go into open attention again. Or they sense that they're uncentred or bracing their muscles unnecessarily, so they let go and come back to balance, allowing their system's innate tendency towards ease and skilfulness to re-establish itself.

For many of us, though, it's not so simple. We've spent so much time being anxious, misusing our attention, bracing and holding ourselves unnecessarily, and moving in ways that contradict our system's innate propensity to organise ease, that these patterns have become ingrained. Over time, chronic muscular tension has reduced our sensory sensitivity and distorted our senses. Unhelpful ways of moving have become embedded in action sequences and habits that take us further and further away from the natural skilfulness and ease that we're capable of. We may even have lost touch with ourselves and our bodies to such an extent that we're not aware of how far from that ease and skilfulness we have strayed.

I sometimes compare this situation to a tangled thread. The things that have gone on in our minds and bodies over many years have caused interlocking, interdependent knots and jams. Unhelpful habits in the way we deal with emotional arousal, use our attention, move and hold ourselves, interact and reinforce each other until it all becomes snarled up in a knot.

Fortunately, though, the mind and body are extraordinarily adaptable and can be changed radically for the better with a little care, commitment and attention. New information and experiences can alter old thought patterns and beliefs. Unhelpful habits can be brought into awareness and unlearned well into old age. An anxious nervous system can be gently encouraged to calm down. Chronically contracted muscles can soften and lengthen again. The accuracy and sensitivity of our senses, and our ability to be gently present to ourselves and our surroundings, can be reawakened. We can discover new ways of moving that are more in tune with the way our system evolved to work. Suppressed and repressed emotions can be resolved and let go of. Gradually the tangle can release, allowing us to return to balance.

A tangled thread may look intimidating but it's not such a big deal if we would only clear a little space and time for it. We investigate what's going on with the tangle and wonder what needs to happen to help loosen it. Carefully and delicately we see if we can ease one of the knots just a little. And then, with no sense of rushing, a little more. And then the next one. And, in time, the next.

This is where Alexander work can come in, helping us to pause and be present for long enough to become aware of our tangle and the things we get up to that cause and sustain it, giving us a chance to consider, understand and make fresh choices that are more in accord with the free and easy way our system evolved to work. We rediscover what it means to find ease, and to move and do things in ways that don't disturb that ease once it's established. Bit by bit things start to let go and return to balance as each jam and knot that loosens makes the next one a little easier.

We'll be exploring this gentle untangling process in the remainder of the book.

Part Four
Coming Home

Chapter Nineteen
Towards Wholeness

So far we've explored how our body, mind and emotions function and interact to support us in the field of gravity and enable us to move and do things. I've suggested that even though the different parts of the Self can work in harmony allowing ease to spontaneously arise in our system, in many of us they often work against each other causing unnecessary discomfort, awkwardness and stress. In this next part of the book we're going to start thinking about how you might go about gently encouraging your system back towards easy, skilful ways of being and moving by making various changes—in awareness and attention, in your relationship with gravity, and in the way you think about moving and going about your life.

As we've seen, change usually involves a bit of a tug-of-war inside us. We may like the idea of making things easier and more pleasant for ourselves and if offered a convincing-sounding way to do so may be willing to give it a go. At the same time we all have some resistance to changing even when we know it would be in our interests. Change takes time and energy which must be diverted from other things, and there's something comforting about the familiarity of what we're used to even if it comes with significant drawbacks. But let's say you've decided to commit to exploring the things I'm suggesting in this book for a while. Three key attitudes, or 'willingnesses', will make all the difference in bringing about the positive results you're hoping for:

1. A willingness to **take time**—by setting time aside to practise, by giving the process of change as long as it takes, and by being willing to be present in the moment as you go about your day.

2. A willingness to experience yourself in ways that may initially feel strange and **unfamiliar**.

3. A willingness to find (at least to begin with) a **teacher** to help you.

Let's look at each of these more closely.

Taking Time

All of us are confronted with a fundamental contradiction. In a sense, the only time we really have is now. We can only experience the actuality of ourselves, each other and the world around us in the present moment. But, simultaneously, anything we want to do or achieve has to involve a process *through* time that requires a relationship with the past, present and future.

In the modern world, our actions and decisions are often driven by the clock. A relentless agenda seems to push us from place to place and from one task to another. Our bodies, on the other hand, have their own sense of time. They want to sleep, wake, eat, stretch, yawn and move at their own pace.*

It's easy for the body's needs and desires to get trampled on in the day-to-day grind of survival and working towards

---

* 'There is mechanical time and there is body time. The first is as rigid and metallic as a massive pendulum of iron . . . The second squirms and wriggles like a bluefish in a bay.' Alan Lightman, *Einstein's Dream*.

our dreams and aspirations. Hopefully by practising the Alexander Technique we'll learn to be kinder to our bodies and to give them more of the time and space they need to be themselves. But still, if we want to do anything worthwhile and function as a member of society we have to engage with the problem of time. We can't give in completely to the pleasures of the moment.

Time to Practise

If you decide to take on board the insights and suggestions I'm offering in this book, it will probably require some shifts in the way you see and understand yourself, and the questioning of some deep-seated assumptions. You may have believed until now, for example, that concentrating makes learning easier, or that 'sitting up straight' and holding yourself in a fixed position is good for you, or that excess muscular tension and the associated pain and discomfort is something which inevitably happens to us as we get older rather than something that we play at least a part in creating and sustaining through our attitudes and actions. But as well as questioning these things, it will also be necessary to learn (or relearn) some subtle but fundamental *skills* to do with how you focus your attention, move, balance and relate to your breath, body and emotions. So, as with learning any skill, you'll need to practise, consistently setting aside short periods of time to gently explore things in a structured way.

Think about how a musician approaches learning their instrument. Every day they pick it up for a while to play scales and exercises, carefully practise the pieces they're working on, do some ear-training and so on. Because it's an important part of their life they also tend to practise at odd moments, picking up the instrument for a minute or two in passing, tapping out rhythms while waiting for the bus, or humming a complex melody while washing up. Practice is something they set aside time for and do willingly because they know it's the only way towards experiencing the rewards of being able to play really well.

In a similar fashion, we'll need to put a chunk of time aside each day—maybe fifteen or twenty minutes—to explore what it means to find ease and take it skilfully into activity. There's lots in the rest of this book about how we might go about this.

Hopefully, as well as setting aside a dedicated chunk of time, we'll take additional odd moments during the day to play with these things too. Perhaps we're about to sit down or stand up from a chair in our usual, rushed way and we think, *No! I'm going to stop, take a bit of time and wonder about what it would take to do this with some delicacy, sensitivity and ease.* Perhaps, waiting at the bus stop, we play with shifting our weight from leg to leg, or with taking a step forwards and back, exploring whether we can stay centred while doing so. Or in the face of a source of anxiety we wonder what it would take to find a little bit of ease and grounded support in that moment.

Sometimes our practice is interesting and absorbing. We're drawn to it, finding all sorts of things to explore and work on. At other times we may find ourselves reluctant or resistant. We get jaded and feel stuck, or even that we're going backwards. It seems that there's so much else that's more important or fun to do. But setting aside time for it is still a valuable commitment. Without ongoing practice we'll never gain sufficient understanding and experience to be able to apply the principles in our life more generally and to experience the rewards, while the regular ongoing engagement with the work acts as a kind of touchstone, reminding us every day that we've decided to pay attention to the way we think, move and do things.

The Time Things Take

One of the non-negotiables in life—which seems obvious, but which many of us nevertheless struggle to fully appreciate—is that things take as long as they take. There's no teleporter to take us down to the shops in an instant, and there's no time machine to get us to the end of a process of learning and change before we've allowed the time that's necessary for those changes to come about.

I once visited a boatbuilder's shed which had 'Good things take time' carved on the lintel over the doors. Having worked as a craftsperson myself, I understand the impulse behind this. Sometimes people want something beautiful and special but they don't want to wait. They want it yesterday. You agree to make it for them but then there is constant hassle. 'Is it ready yet? When will it be ready? Why is it taking so long?'

Ideally one is able to put these demands to one side, but it can become uncomfortable. If you give in, though, you'll invariably start to rush, and sooner or later you will make a mistake. It might not be the end of the world, but the beautiful thing is marred nonetheless. It's not quite what it could be. In the end I had 'Good things take time' embroidered on my overalls so that when people visited the workshop they would get the message!

If you decide to take the ideas in this book seriously, you'll be working to change action sequences and habits that have built up over many years. This takes time, because habits and action sequences are not only formed but *modified* through repetition. It's not difficult. All we have to do is repeatedly catch ourselves in the act, pause, and make a different choice. But because many of the things we hope to change are rather subtle, and have been ingrained over many years, and because we need to discover and refine new action sequences and fresh ways of responding to replace them, it doesn't happen overnight. We fall into our old ways again and again. But if we keep making more beneficial choices, those old ways gradually start to loosen their hold. In the end, it becomes less comfortable and natural to respond in the old way than in the new ones we've discovered.

In addition to this gradual change in our habits and ways of doing things, there's also a process of inner reflection and change that needs to happen as we gently question some of our long-standing ideas and attitudes towards ourselves, our goals and the ways we go about things. This, too, takes time. It takes time for new understandings to clarify and settle. Physical changes will also need to happen in the body to enable and support new ways of being and acting in the world. It takes time for muscles that have been chronically tightened to get used to letting go and returning to their proper length. Conversely, muscles that have been chronically underused due to other muscles overworking may need time to gradually strengthen so that they can play their proper role throughout the day. And it takes time for stress-related chemicals and hormones that have built up in our body over many years to be flushed away as our system calms and quietens down, and for our system to let go of other accumulated effects of stress and tension and come back to balance.

Some people are naturally quite patient. They don't mind taking as long as it takes to get where they are going. Others have more of a tendency to rush and be in a hurry. I can relate to this! It's a difficult habit to let go of. At times we may find our pace of progress tiresomely slow and want to obsessively push things along. But this is counterproductive. The rushing, anxiety and concentration that go along with the pushing make us tighten and brace, contradicting the changes we want. Paradoxically, it makes it all take longer.

We may even be tempted to give up in frustration at how long it's taking and try some other practice or solution instead. Some people spend years jumping from practice to practice, never giving anything they do the chance to settle and make a significant difference. In life, though, there don't tend to be magic bullets to solve our problems. Worthwhile things take a bit of commitment and consistency. They take the time that they take, and the indispensable key to real, worthwhile change is agreeing to give it to them.

Time and the Present Moment

So far we've considered time in the sense of its passage—putting aside regular time to practise, and allowing sufficient time for positive change to come about. But to make use in our lives of what we're discovering in our practice, we also need to be taking time in the sense of being present in the moment—less on autopilot, less controlled by habit, less lost in our heads and more aware of where we are and what we're doing right now.

We've already seen that presence is an essential quality of ease. Sometimes it arises spontaneously on its own.

Perhaps you're reading a book late at night, lost in the author's imaginary world, when you hear an unexpected creak at the bottom of the stairs. Instantly, without thinking about it or trying, you're right there in the room, listening. Or you may be in a beautiful place or doing something you enjoy or are deeply interested in and presence arises quite simply and naturally on its own.

Often, though, we need to *choose* to be present. We notice we've become lost in our thoughts, hopes, plans and fears, and have lost contact with our senses and the world around us, and we make the simple choice to come back.

Of course, reflection, dreams and reverie are important parts of being human too. It's alright to be lost in our minds and imaginations at times. But generally, when we notice we're not really here it's good to choose to return. Try it now! Put the book to one side and look around you. What is there to see? What quality of light and shade? What sounds are there? And what is going on with your body—your limbs, your orientation in space, tension or ease in your musculature, sensations of warmth and cold and the surface of your skin?

Perhaps it sounds like it might be hard work, or even a bit of a chore, to choose to be present as much as possible as we go about our lives, but really it's a lovely thing. It puts us in touch with the *actual* life we're living—the only one we have, *this* one that is only ever happening now—while at the same time taking us off autopilot, giving us the chance to make the sort of choices that lead to comfort, freedom and ease in ourselves, our actions and our relationships.

This ongoing choice to be present in the moment is not the same thing as practising. Think about the musician again. They know the difference between practising and playing. When they practise they slow things down or break them up, focusing on a particular area, working deliberately and intelligently with a view to improvement. When they *play*, however, they put that considered deliberateness aside and just make music. At those times they're not working towards getting better—they're vibrantly in the moment with their instrument, the music and themselves, just as they are. Whatever they've practised has become a reliable resource for them to draw on.

We can approach ease and skilfulness like this too. As we discover more about these things through our practice, we increasingly find that we can apply this understanding to whatever we're doing as we go about our lives making everything easier and more enjoyable. But we can only do this if we're here in the moment, present to ourselves and the world around us.

Experiencing the New

The second of the essential key attitudes I mentioned is a willingness to experience yourself in ways that feel strange and unfamiliar.

Try crossing your arms and legs, then pausing and crossing them the other way. Most likely the second way feels a bit odd and unnatural and you wouldn't want to stay like that for very long. Over time, our habits often come to feel natural, normal and right—as if they're intrinsic, unchangeable aspects of ourselves rather than ways of being and acting which we adopted for various reasons at specific points in the past. Do you remember the chap in the first chapter who, even though he could see the pain, discomfort and stress caused by a lifetime of chronic, driven busyness, still found that, when push came to shove, he didn't want to change after all? It was more important to him to experience himself in his familiar way than it was to reduce the tension and pain it was causing him.

So if you're interested in exploring the changes I'm suggesting in this book, you must be willing to allow yourself to feel strange and unfamiliar sometimes. These feelings of unfamiliarity can take several forms. First, we can experience changes in our beliefs and attitudes. For example, if we're like the man described above we may decide, after some reflection, that it would be better for us to go about things in a gentler, less busy and driven way. This can be disconcerting to begin with if our self-image is of being a busy person whom others depend on, or if we believe that our survival or important life goals depend on our driven mindset. Or, in contrast, we may be a rather more lackadaisical, unfocused person and decide that we'll benefit from bringing a bit more structure, energy and attention to what we're doing. This may challenge our self-image and sense of ourselves as a chilled person who goes with the flow.

Second, we will need to experience ourselves differently at a physical level too. As we learn to stop bracing ourselves for stabilisation and support, and allow ourselves a more dynamic way of being, our felt sense of how our body is put together changes. We may begin to sit, stand and do things in ways that feel strange and crooked to begin with. We may feel so strange that initially we think we could never allow ourselves to be seen in public in such a state!

Fortunately, although these sorts of changes can feel unsettling, the feeling generally passes quite quickly. Humans are adaptable. We can adjust to new ways of experiencing ourselves, particularly when we discover after a while how much easier, lighter and more effective they are. We find that, far from making people think we look odd, the strange new way of moving we've discovered, attracts no notice—or even that people like it or are envious of it. Or we find that we're becoming more effective in spite of rushing around less. We notice that we're doing things better, with more consideration, care and attention.

As we become comfortable with this evolving version of ourselves, we find that many habits we were once so attached to and identified with were only impediments. What at first seems very odd comes to seem as much like 'us' as the old pattern did. In fact it often comes to feel *more* like us, because to get there we removed layers of unnecessary tension, stress and effort which obscured our true nature.

Working with a Teacher

As you continue through this book you may be wondering if you need a teacher to really understand and put into practice what you're reading. It's a good question. I'd say that although, in theory, you may be able to get some of the benefits working entirely on your own, in practice you probably won't get too far without someone to help you, at least at the beginning.

While this work isn't exactly difficult, it's rather *subtle*. It's easy to misinterpret, half understand or miss the point of the words on the page in one way or another, or to devalue an essential bit of advice or information without realising you're doing so. A teacher can help you avoid this.

Many years ago, I spent some time learning to build boats. The first stage was an intensive three-month course in using hand tools. I was experienced with tools already in a self-taught sort of way. I confess I even wondered whether I needed to be in the class at all. One early exercise involved making a scarf joint. Scarf joints are where you make a long piece of timber from two shorter ones by cutting and planing a diagonal face at one end of each piece and glueing them together. For the joint to be strong and last as long as possible, each diagonal face has to be totally flat, kissing the other cleanly, without any gaps or wobbles so there's the maximum possible surface for the glue to stick to. This is particularly important in boatbuilding to prevent any ingress of water into the joint.

We were told to plane this diagonal face on each piece, checking both parts carefully with a straight edge for any bumps or dips. When we thought our work was good enough, we were to ask an instructor to check before we glued the parts together. All of us worked away for a while, checking for flatness as carefully as we could, and then put up our hands expecting to be told to go ahead and glue up. But, without exception, when the instructor came over to each of us he'd find a tiny bump we had missed. He would lay the straight edge on the spot and show us the little wobble. So we went back to work, checked again, called him over again, and the same thing happened.

And again. And again.

It started to freak us out! No matter how carefully we checked, we were unable to see the problems until they were pointed out to us.

We asked the teacher what was going on. 'You don't see what you don't want to see,' he replied. 'If you see the problem you have to do more work, and you don't like working, so you unconsciously choose not to see it.'

Eventually our brains adjusted and we started to see the tiny bumps and dips for ourselves. Our perception had been permanently expanded by being shown what we didn't want to see.

None of us know what we don't know, and—by definition—we can't see our own blind spots. So one of the most helpful things a teacher can do for us is to *point out*, showing us things we'd otherwise unconsciously resist seeing for ourselves.

Often it seems rather quiet in an Alexander lesson. Much of the time will likely be spent quietly standing, sitting, lying and making simple movements such as standing up and sitting down, reaching or walking. It's a different pace to everyday life. The teacher may have their hands on the student for some of this time, communicating a sense of calmness and quiet. A good teacher uses their own state of being to help calm your nervous system, encouraging stuck vicious circles of over-arousal, endgaining and effortfulness to ease and let go. They may also use their hands to guide you into unfamiliar patterns of movement, helping to delicately dissolve blocks and resistances and encouraging you to experience yourself in a new way. In the process, they can help you notice habits and subtle proprioceptive signals that are easy to miss on your own. If you habitually hold yourself in crooked or misaligned ways which you have come to experience as upright and aligned, a teacher can use their hands to help you regain an accurate sense of yourself. It would likely take much longer for you to experience this on your own because it can feel so strange and wrong to begin with. A new experience of balance may even feel *dangerous*, as if you might fall, even if you're actually now more stable than you were before. It can be hard to believe that something that feels out of balance is safe. Usually, though, it only takes a bit of support and reassurance from the teacher (together with the experience that you don't, in fact, fall over) for this illusion to begin to naturally correct itself.

A teacher can also help you *keep going*. All of us have limited time and many competing priorities, and any worthwhile learning process has periods when we seem stuck, or even like we're going backwards. If you're working away at something on your own and it seems you're not getting anywhere, it's likely that sooner or later—unless you're very unusually strong-willed and persistent—you will give up. A teacher can keep you on track, offering encouragement while sharing their knowledge and experience of the journey. They help you avoid common beginner's mistakes, misunderstandings and dead-ends, enabling you to experience the benefits much sooner, which helps to give you the motivation to continue.

Though it might seem like it would be saving time and money to teach yourself, it's often a false economy. A teacher *saves* you time. In terms of the health and other benefits that can come with the work, they'll often save you money too, in the long run. If you're drawn to exploring the ideas in this book and putting them into practice, I strongly suggest that, if you don't already have one, you find a teacher to accompany you on the journey for a while.

Chapter Twenty
Pausing to Find Ease

We've seen that many of us find it difficult to access a state of quiet ease in ourselves and to move freely and skilfully in activity. But even someone who is generally very open, free and well-coordinated can become unsettled in the daily ebb and flow of their lives. Perhaps due to a sudden shock or distraction, stress, tiredness or a moment of clumsiness or imbalance, they get out of kilter causing them to brace and tighten. So, whatever our starting point, the ability to find ease, and to recover it again when it is lost, is an essential human ability.

In principle, finding ease is a simple, natural thing. After all, our system *wants* to manifest ease. Ease is its default state which establishes itself as soon as the conditions are right. We don't need to be busily doing things to find ease. We simply need to choose to be present and centred while *not doing* anything that gets in its way (we'll be talking a lot more about this business of 'not doing' in the next few chapters).

In the end, finding ease can become so simple and accessible that it can happen in a heartbeat—in the space between two footsteps, in the shifting of weight as we move our hands around the piano, in the momentary pause as we respond to our dance partner's impetus into movement, or between deciding to reach out for the dishes and extending our arms to lift them from the water. Even amid movement and activity it's possible to allow our system to settle and return to ease as and when we need to.

Hopefully you'll be able to access ease in the moment like this for yourself before too long. But suppose you're new to these ideas. You may be caught in a bit of a tangle of habits and unreliable sensory appreciation that makes it unrealistic to expect to be able to do so just yet. So to begin with, you'll need to give yourself and your nervous system a bit of extra time to make the transition to ease. You'll need to consciously interrupt your stream of habitual thought and activity by gently **pausing** and coming to rest.

When I talk about pausing like this, I'm not thinking about a fierce, forced sort of pause like slamming on the brakes. Nor am I talking about the sort of pause we make reluctantly, holding ourselves on tenterhooks just waiting for the chance to get going again. Rather, I'm talking about a generous, whole-hearted sort of pause—a decision to really, genuinely stop and give yourself some time to consider, be curious and wonder about the state you're in and what you're up to.

So let's say you've decided to pause with a general intention to settle and find a bit of ease in yourself. How can you go about creating the conditions necessary to enable that ease to manifest? What would it be helpful to be considering and to be curious *about*?

The seven qualities of ease that we met earlier (*quietness, presence, openness, freedom, centredness, dynamic stabilisation and grounded support*) can help us with this, giving us a useful framework to work within and prompting and guiding our explorations. Here are seven questions based on those qualities to get you started:

1. Are you inwardly **quiet**? Or are you mentally churning, full of thoughts and worries about the past and future, or busily trying to fix some worrying pain or discomfort through tension, holding and effort?

   Can you be open to the idea of putting any compulsive thoughts, worries and busy attempts to fix yourself aside for a little while, deciding instead to make some space to quieten down, settle and find some ease?

2. Are you **present**—really *here*, now, in this moment? Or are you absent and distracted, lost in your thoughts or otherwise disconnected from your sense of yourself and your surroundings?

   Perhaps you could make a simple decision to be here—to gently land in yourself, your senses and the world around you.

3. Is there a gentle **openness** in your field of attention, and particularly in your visual field, or are you concentrating, your awareness narrowed down, your eyes staring and intent, your head fixed rigidly on your shoulders?

   Perhaps you could choose to stop with all the intentness allowing your awareness of yourself and your surroundings to broaden, bringing in all of your senses, leaving your eyes and head free to move as they will.

4. Is there unbraced **freedom** throughout the joints of your structure, and particularly in your breath? Or are you bracing your joints, or holding and constricting your breathing in your belly or across the width of your ribcage, preventing each breath from coming and going lightly and easily in its own way?

   Perhaps you could choose to simply stop doing these things.

These first four questions are always applicable, even if we're lying down completely supported by the ground. But the last three become relevant only when we're upright and needing active support from our muscles in the field of gravity.

5. Are you **centred** with your weight placed somewhere close to the middle of your base of support? Or is it held *off*-centre, causing muscles in your feet and legs to brace for security?

   Perhaps you could take a moment to find your centre, gently shifting your weight around until it arrives in that small, sensitive zone where your joints and breath spontaneously free up a little.

6. Is your body alive with the subtle, spontaneous movements of **dynamic stabilisation**? Or are you fixing and holding yourself to stay upright in the field of gravity?

   Perhaps you can let things delicately move as they want to, allowing your body to dynamically self-organise as it finds balance and support in its own way.

7. Are you in a state of **grounded support**, your weight resting freely and easily on the Earth beneath you? Or are you collapsed, or pulling yourself down, or pulling up and away, disconnecting from the ground?

   Perhaps you can let your weight rest lightly on the ground and allow dynamic support to release upwards, leaving your spine free to naturally adopt its full, unforced length and your head to balance freely and easily on top.

So long as you are in a reasonably calm state to begin with, these simple wonderings can be sufficient to enable your system to settle and return to ease.

Sometimes, though—and particularly when we're just starting out with these explorations—it doesn't seem nearly as easy and straightforward as I've made it sound here. In the next chapter we're going to look at why this is so often the case, before going on to learn more about not doing, and about a simple practice called **not-this-not-that** which offers us a simple, elegant way through the difficulty.

Chapter Twenty-One

Difficulties with Ease

Imagine someone coming for their first Alexander lesson. Let's say that generally things have been going well enough for them in their lives so far. They aren't carrying significant physical injuries. They don't have a history of overwhelmingly painful emotional experiences or trauma. Their life isn't excessively difficult or stressful at a practical level. On the whole, things are OK. Nevertheless, over the years they've become rather tense and uncomfortable in themselves and have noticed themselves becoming a little held and awkward in their activities. Perhaps they've noticed they don't move as freely and easily as they would like, or they're experiencing aches, pains and emotional stress which seem to be related to excess physical tension or lack of muscular support. Maybe they feel this is limiting the ease and skilfulness they can bring to activities they enjoy or depend on for their livelihood.

Let's imagine that, after talking things over for a while, the teacher suggests that this student takes a moment or two to pause—just to be sitting or standing quietly for a while, being open and present, allowing their breath to move freely, gently stopping with any intentness, concentration or muscular bracing that they're doing, giving their system a chance to settle and self-organise in an easy, dynamic way.

Although the student will certainly try to do what's

being asked of them, the results are likely to be quite different from the quiet, present, open state the teacher is pointing to. Despite their attempts to put the teacher's suggestions into practice, their nervous system is likely to remain rather over-activated and on edge. Quite possibly they'll still be lost in their head, distracted or tuned out. Their field of attention will remain fixed and narrow, their breathing somewhat tight and restricted, their structure braced for stability.

It may even seem that not only is the student failing to put the teacher's suggestions into practice, but that these suggestions are actually *exacerbating* these tensions in their system. If the teacher suggests that they be a little less intent, the person spaces out and dissociates or gets further mired in concentration and effortfulness. If it's suggested that they allow their breath to move freely, or stop holding and bracing themselves so that their system a chance to release into dynamic freedom and ease, they actually hold their breath and tighten and brace further. The *exact opposite* of what is being asked for is happening! Moreover, although the teacher can see this easily, the student is often completely unaware that it's happening. What's going on?

Generally, it's a few specific things that are causing the difficulty:

- Anxiousness about the learning process
- Strength of habit
- Unreliable sensory appreciation
- The challenge of not doing

In the rest of this chapter we're going to look at these more closely.

Anxiousness About the Learning Process

We may or may not be worried about things that are going on in our lives more generally, but when we start deliberately engaging in a learning process aimed at changing long-standing habits and ways of being, some level of anxiousness is often evoked by the learning process itself. We saw earlier that learning—either on our own or in a lesson with a teacher—is, for many people, associated with unpleasant prior experiences which may have included being pressured, judged and shamed, or simply failing to come up to our own or others' expected standards. If this is the case, being in a learning situation can make us subtly or obviously anxious, causing spontaneous concentration, constricted breathing, and muscular bracing strong enough to override anything more positive that we'd like to happen. We can easily get caught in a seemingly no-win situation—a vicious circle—in which our anxious desire to make positive changes and 'get it right' triggers the very same patterns of anxiety, concentration and muscular tension which created the state we are now hoping to change.

Strength of Habit

Another thing that can interfere with finding ease is the strength of our current unhelpful habits. They may have become so strong and ingrained that even if we momentarily lay them aside they immediately get triggered again. For example, I may have such a strong habit of concentrating when I'm trying to do something which I believe is difficult that, even if I'm able to stop concentrating for a moment, some other aspect of the learning process will immediately re-trigger it. Or I may have developed so many habitual ways of bracing and holding myself that even if I stop doing one of them, another immediately takes its place.

Unreliable Sensory Appreciation

We saw earlier that it's likely that our sense of ourselves has become inaccurate. The sensory feedback which tells us whether we're upright, how our body parts are aligned, how we're moving, and how much effort is needed to move and support our structure, doesn't necessarily accord with the way things actually are.

Not only that, but our familiar ways of being and moving will often have come to feel normal, familiar and 'right' even when they're unhelpful or harmful. This feeling of normality can get in the way of change. Even though our system may be wanting to spontaneously adopt a healthier way of organising itself, it can be difficult for us give it permission to so if that way feels unfamiliar, strange or wrong.

The Challenge of Not Doing

We've also seen that, because ease arises in our system spontaneously rather than being produced directly by our voluntary efforts, finding it is mostly about *not* doing things rather than about doing them. We need to stop interfering and get out of its way. But many of us are simply not used to going about things like this. We have an effortful, doing-based approach to life which seems so obviously right to us—and that is so long-practised and culturally encouraged—that we can't quite accept it's part of the problem. We can't quite believe that just by getting out of the way and giving our system a bit of space and time to respond, the relaxed state of dynamic ease we hope for will come about naturally on its own. Surely (we secretly think) we'll need to help it along just a *little* bit—a tiny nudge here, a little holding and bracing there. Even if we understand the argument intellectually, we still don't quite get, deep down, that choosing *not* to do things will be sufficient to lead to worthwhile positive change. In fact we may have become so used to responding to every challenge we meet by doing something that the ability to *not* do has become unfamiliar and difficult to access, even if we'd like to. We're completely out of touch with what it means.

This business of not doing is right at the heart of our problem. In the next couple of chapters we're going to learn more about it. First I'm going to tell you about three different *kinds* of not doing, and then I'll introduce you to a practice that I call **not-this-not-that**, which offers a simple but profound approach to accessing not doing for yourself.

Chapter Twenty-Two
Not Doing

All you want is a little bit of nothing.
—MARJORIE BARSTOW, Aphorisms

We've seen that the idea of doing something to get what we want, to make changes in ourselves or to solve a problem is very familiar and comfortable for most of us. It tends to be the default way we approach things. But we've also begun to see that there's another, more subtle approach, which is to wonder what we might be up to that's causing the problem or getting in the way of what we want, and to remove those things by making wise **negative choices**. There are three types of negative choice we can make:

1. We can **stop doing** something that is *already going on*. Perhaps we notice we're concentrating or rigidly sitting up straight, and we simply decide to stop doing it.

2. We can **say no** to unhelpful habits and responses *as they arise* in us—noticing unhelpful things we're *about* to do or that are *about* to happen (such as the impulse to concentrate, or to use an unintegrated movement pattern, or to brace for support, or to hold our breath), and choosing not to do them *at all*.

3. We can choose to **allow** healthy natural processes (such as the delicate spontaneous movements of breathing and of dynamic stabilisation and support) to unfold freely as they will.

Let's think further about these three types of not doing.

Stopping Doing

Stopping doing is about things we're *already* up to, or which are *already* going on. Perhaps I'm standing with my knees locked, or I'm effortfully bracing myself to 'sit up straight'. Or I might notice that I'm concentrating, intently narrowing my field of attention and fixing my eyes and head. Or perhaps I'm ungrounding myself, pulling my breastbone and the arches of my feet up away from the floor. In each of these cases it would be helpful to simply stop doing those things.

It's essential to understand that I'm not talking here about relaxing in the sense of trying to release tight and tense muscles. Although this seems like an obvious thing to try to do if we feel tense, it's not very effective because it works against the way our voluntary systems for moving and controlling our body evolved to work. Our muscles exist not for their own sake but for the sake of the joints and body parts that they support and move. We're not supposed to control muscles directly. When we want to raise our arms we don't need to think about the muscles involved and making them contract or relax—we ask our arms to go up and up they go! That's how the system works, and it makes perfect sense. So rather than trying to relax tense muscles directly, it's much more helpful to notice whatever mental decision or impulse is *behind* any bracing and holding that's going on, and simply decide to stop doing it. The muscles involved will take care of themselves in their own way.

Saying No

Saying no is another kind of negative choice. Rather than stopping something that is already going on, it involves deciding to withhold consent from something that is *about* to happen so that it doesn't even get going in the first place.[*]

One set of things we can learn to say no to is habits. I might notice, for example, that I'm about to become intent and concentrate—as is my habit. Or I might see, as I sit on my chair, that I'm about to sit up rigidly straight as I usually do. Or in getting up from the chair I might notice that I'm about to effortfully haul and push myself up in my habitual fashion. Or when playing the piano I might see that I'm about to pound into the keybed with my fingers as I play a chord.

If I become aware of these habitual impulses as they arise, I then have the chance to choose not to go with them—to withhold consent—opening up a space in which there is the possibility of responding to the situation differently.

As well as saying no to habits, we may in time find that we can begin to gently say no to some of the physical manifestations of our emotional responses, too. If something anxious-making happens, for example, and I realise that my musculature and breath are about to tighten in response, I can say to myself, *Actually, no, I don't think I'll respond that way. I'd prefer to stay open and free today.* Gradually we find that we're beginning to be able to gently nip these kinds of responses in the bud, at least some of the time.

---

[*] F.M. Alexander, drawing on the scientific terminology of his day, called saying no 'inhibition'. I'm not keen on this though, because it comes with unhelpful connotations—few of us would aspire to be 'inhibited'! So I'll stick with 'saying no', which points more directly to the clear, gentle quality of negative decision I'm talking about.

Intriguingly, by saying no to the physical part of the response we also influence the feeling because they're opposite sides of the same coin. You can't have one without the other. So learning to say no can be a powerful tool to help us manage our emotions.

It's important to be clear that saying no to something isn't at all the same thing as suppressing it. It's not that the thing is still wanting to happen under the surface, and we're blocking it or applying muscular tension to cover it up. That would be counterproductive. Rather, we are making a simple, clear choice to not go with the impulse *at all*.

Allowing

The third type of negative choice I want to consider is to *allow*—choosing to get out of the way of healthy spontaneous processes and movements so they can establish themselves and continue without interference. I might allow my breath to move freely, for example, letting it self-regulate and quietly do its thing. Or I might allow my system to organise the delicate adjustments and movements associated with dynamic stabilisation, balance and support. Or I might choose to stop pulling down and contracting my torso, neck and head, allowing my spine to spontaneously release into its full, unforced length.

You can probably see that allowing something to happen often requires both stopping doing and saying no—we need to get out of the way and then stay out of the way! But at the same time, allowing is phenomenologically distinct. We experience it as its own thing, born specifically from the desire to let some process or movement establish itself and continue. We can stop doing something or say no to a single impulse and be done with it. Allowing, on the other hand, is about a gentle *ongoing* refusal to interfere with some healthy spontaneous process that wants to unfold through time.

The Four Buttons

It's vital to realise that these three negative abilities aren't just another, more subtle form of doing. They're something else entirely, arising from different processes in the brain.

I sometimes joke with my students and tell them that they have four buttons inside their heads. First, there's the 'do' button. It is large, bright red, plastic and is right in front of them. It has a big label on it that says 'press me'. It looks like the sort of button that would make stuff happen—like it would be a good button to press in an emergency. We're all very familiar with the 'do' button.

But we also have three smaller and more delicate, mother-of-pearl buttons. They're beautifully crafted, tucked away in a quiet room that we rarely go into anymore, covered in a thick layer of dust. We may have completely forgotten that this room exists. If our house is rather large and rambling we may not even be able to find the room, let alone the buttons. But if you were to stumble upon them, you would see that each one has, beautifully engraved in a fine font, its own small label:

'Stop doing'

'Say no'

'Allow'

They look like the sort of buttons you wouldn't want to be in a rush with. If you were to press them at all, you would probably be inclined to do so with a degree of reverence and care.

There's nothing inherently wrong with the 'do' button—it's necessary and useful. The trouble is that it's so big and tempting, and we're so used to pressing it, that we get into the habit of going for it whenever we meet any challenge at all—even when it would be far better to think about pressing the 'stop doing', 'say no' or 'allow' button instead. Over and over again we jab at that tempting bright red button. In fact for many of us, taking positive action has become such a deeply embedded habit that even the wish to make a negative decision instead—to stop doing something, to say no to a habit or response, or to allow something to happen—triggers even more desperate stabs at the 'do' button.

All of our habitual effortfulness ends up in our Alexander practice! We try so hard to not concentrate that we concentrate even more in the attempt. We tighten our braced joints even as we attempt to stop doing so. In the hope of allowing our breath to do its own thing we subtly or not-so-subtly interfere with it. We may even believe that these attempts are successful when in fact we're just using the 'do' button to suppress and hold back the things we hoped to *not* do.

This tendency to default to doing even as we intend to not do is exacerbated by an anxious, stressed and over-stimulated nervous system. The changes in the brain that happen when we're anxious make us become oriented towards action and doing. So even a little bit of momentary anxiousness makes it more difficult for us to connect with our innate ability to pause, calmly consider and choose to stop doing, say no, or allow, putting those three delicate buttons even further out of reach. The harder we try the more difficult we make it, and the more we worry about how difficult it seems to be, the worse it gets. It's as if, while teasing away to ease a tangled thread, we find in our eagerness that we're tugging at it in a rather impatient, forceful way, making matters worse. Out of anxiousness, impatience or a lack of sensitivity we're tightening the knot rather than loosening it.

Somehow we need to rediscover what it means to access those three delicate not-doing buttons, despite the temptation of that bright, compelling 'do' button. And, at the same time, we need to address the seemingly no-win situation that—for many of us—anxiousness about learning to do this tends to make it harder still, encouraging the very same tension, stress and overdoing that we hope to let go of.

Fortunately, there's a simple but profound answer to this puzzle. We'll find out about it in the next chapter.

Chapter Twenty-Three
Not-This-Not-That

When you stop doing the wrong thing, the right thing does itself.
—F.M. Alexander, attrib.

I wonder if you've heard of a Hindu meditation practice called neti-neti? Neti-neti means 'not this, not that'. It aims to help one approach God, or ultimate reality (or whatever you want to call that ineffable ground of being), not through trying to find out what it *is* but by giving attention to what it is *not*. Whatever that mysterious, unknown, timeless thing is, the reasoning goes, it must be completely beyond our limited human concerns, thoughts and experiences—something entirely other than our limited, time-bound, fragmented everyday selves. And so because anything we might do to try and reach it, experience it or hold on to it can come only from that limited everyday self, all our attempts are not only 'not it', but actively contradict and obscure it.

If something is beyond what we know, and is contradicted and obscured by anything we might do to pursue it directly, then we can only approach it *indirectly*, by beginning to notice what it is *not*—which includes all our misguided attempts to find it. As we begin to understand that 'it' cannot possibly be 'this' or 'that'—when all that has been negated and disavowed—we may find that this leaves a space for that unknown, ineffable thing to enter.

Though very simple, this is a profound philosophy and practice, and the idea behind it is helpful for us too, because we have a similar problem to the meditator. We too are interested in finding a state (ease) that may be unfamiliar and which is always fresh and new—never quite the same from moment to moment—and which has to come about on its own because any attempt to do something to get it will only contradict it and get in its way. Our only viable course is to not do anything that prevents it or interferes with it so it has a chance to manifest on its own.

But, as we've seen, this can be challenging because many of us no longer know what it means to not do. We've lost contact with those three vital negative abilities—stopping doing, saying no and allowing. We tend to reflexively reach for the 'do' button whenever we have a problem to solve, even if it's counterproductive. The harder we try to find the answer, the further away we push it.

Using the idea behind neti-neti (not-this-not-that) can help us with all these problems and contradictions. Rather than going round and round trying effortfully to bring about ease without even really knowing what it is, we can instead start to gently notice, as honestly as we can, what is going on in us that gets in the way of the qualities of ease manifesting in us—*including all our unhelpful attempts to bring them about.*

Take the quality of openness, for example. Imagine I notice that, rather than allowing my field of attention to be open and free, I'm concentrating—my eyes fixed and staring, my visual field narrowed down. Let's say I decide to try to stop being so intent. And yet I notice that what actually happens in response to these attempts is that I get rather busy thinking about what it might take to bring such a happy state of affairs about, and worrying about whether I'm getting it right. I notice that I get a little anxious about it all, that my musculature braces slightly, and I hold my breath a little. If I'm honest with myself, I may even notice that I'm concentrating a little *harder*. So I can be quite clear about one thing at least—*that's not it!* Perhaps I believed that the things I was thinking and doing would be helpful, but with observation and reflection I see that they're taking me further from openness rather than closer to it. I may not know what is needed—what it would actually mean to stop with all that intentness—but I can at least be sure it's not this active, distracted, over-intent thing that I'm up to.

Or maybe I notice that my breath is moving quite tightly and shallowly high up in my chest, and so I think about allowing my belly and ribcage to move freely so that each breath can go easily in and out in its own way. But then I notice I'm putting quite a lot of effort into my attempts to put this idea into practice. I start concentrating, my eyes fixing and my visual field narrowing. I'm subtly bracing my legs and pelvis. Perhaps I find that, in trying to give my belly and ribcage permission to move, I'm actually constricting and controlling my breath a little *more* rather than leaving it free to do its own thing. So I can at least be sure that even if I don't know what it's like to allow my breath to be free, these particular things I am up to in my attempts to do so are *not* it. Once again, my efforts are taking me further from ease, not closer to it.

Or perhaps I notice I'm rather effortfully standing up straight, and think that it would be good to stop holding myself so rigidly, giving my system a chance to manifest a bit of sensitive, alive, dynamic stabilisation instead. But I find that, in response to this idea, I concentrate, or hold my breath, or brace myself in some new way, or let go into a slumpy collapse, or do some other thing that has nothing to do with ease. Yet again, I can be sure that whatever the way is, it's not *this* way!

To begin with, as we play this gentle game with ourselves, we'll probably be so out of touch with our bodies and nervous systems that it will be difficult to spot what we're up to. We may not yet be sensitive enough to be aware of all the various ways we brace our structure to stay upright, or how we tune out from our surroundings and bodily sensations, or concentrate and subtly hold our breath.

But not to worry! Just to be curious and noticing *any* of this is progress. At least we're giving ourselves a *chance* to become more conscious and in touch with ourselves and with the games we play in the pursuit of ease. If we stay with it, gently exploring it for a little while every day, and at odd moments throughout the day, then after a time we'll begin to become more sensitive to it all. We'll begin to notice we've tightened and braced for support even though we meant the opposite to happen. We'll see how we are efforting in our pursuit of effortlessness. We'll begin to notice how, in response to our wish to be quietly present, openly aware and free, we tighten, brace, concentrate, become over-intent and hold and restrict our breathing. We're beginning to be in *actual contact* with the unhelpful things we do which get in the way of the very thing we're hoping to bring about by doing them.

As we start to see these things (I mean *really* see them—not just intellectually as an idea, but actually observing them unfolding in ourselves), the negative choices we need begin to be revealed as the only ones left, because everything else has been seen to be counterproductive, and discounted. More and more we find we can choose to gently stop with our unhelpful holdings, bracings and fixings and allow a bit more freedom and ease into our structure. And, more than this, we find that we're beginning to notice unhelpful habits and responses *as they arise in us*: at first after they've already happened, then as they're actually happening, then just as they're arising, and finally as they're *about* to happen. And increasingly we find that we can choose to gently say no to these responses before they even get going. More and more we find we can leave our body's healthy, natural, spontaneous processes alone, allowing the breath to do its thing, allowing our attention to freely and openly follow our interest, allowing our neuromuscular system to dynamically stabilise, balance and find support without us trying to help it along.

In time, as our braced musculature begins to free up a little, we become more open and sensitive to ourselves and our surroundings. Our sense of our structure and how it's put together and moves becomes more accurate, feeding into our system's increasing capacity for healthy, spontaneous organisation. Round and round we go—gently and patiently circling the problem, dipping in, dipping out, coming in close to this or that aspect of the whole, then pulling back to see the big picture, wondering, exploring and learning. Gradually, our vicious circle becomes a virtuous one. Bit by bit our tangle loosens. We start to experience ourselves in a new way.

I can't emphasise enough the quiet patience we need to bring to all this! It takes a gentle wondering quality—a *genuine* curiousness about what creates ease, and about what arises in ourselves in response to our wish to be at ease. Like growing a flower, you can't force it to open. All you can do is take care of it, ensure it has enough water (not too much) and plenty of warmth and light (again, not too much) and be patient. It will open in its own time. There's no deadline. It's not a race. It's not something you can get by trying. Ease arises when we *stop* trying—when we see effort, concentration, bracing, tightening and imbalance for what they are, and when we understand what they do to us and realise, clearly, simply and unequivocally, that we don't need to go that way anymore.

A Teacher's Help

In truth I've sometimes winced a little while I've been writing this chapter, because although I can give you an indication, I can't show you with words what it's really like to explore in the way I'm suggesting. I can't give you a true *sense* of it—a real appreciation of the care and delicacy that one needs to bring to this process of learning, discovery and change. It's so easy to get the wrong end of the stick without realising it. Despite our best intentions, it's all too easy to bring a rather over-intent, over-anxious energy to it, even if we're determined not to. Our unhelpful habits may be so deeply embedded that they get triggered whichever way we turn. Impatience, endgaining, concentration, bracing and interference may have come to seem so normal to us that they can be difficult to see through on our own.

This can particularly be the case if our motivation for exploring the Alexander Technique is a desire to relieve some distressing problem. Perhaps we're in pain and hoping the Technique will improve things for us. Maybe we're chronically anxious and stressed and looking for relief. Rather than being able to explore in the curious and gentle spirit I'm suggesting, we're constantly breaking off to check in on our problem and see whether what we're doing is working.

Is the pain still there?

Isn't it better yet?

Is it even a little better?

*Will it **ever** get better?*

Will I ever be pain-free and relaxed again?

Might I even have to stop work or change my career?

Cascades of anxiousness are triggered every time we check in on our symptoms like this. And the more anxious we get, the more we get caught in the vicious circle, and the more difficult it all becomes.

A skilled teacher can be so helpful here.

Sometimes when I'm teaching, I'll gently point out the contradictory responses that can arise as a result of a student's earnest hopes for change.

'Did you notice that you started concentrating when I suggested you think about quietening down?'

'Did you see your breath tightened when I suggested allowing your attention to be a little more open to yourself and the world around you?'

'Although we were thinking about allowing freedom and ease just then, did you notice that actually you tensed up and disconnected from the floor?'

Or I might approach it the other way around.

'There!' I'll say as their system spontaneously releases into easy, dynamic support. Or 'Mmmm!' as their attention releases from a rather tight, unhappy, concentrated state into an open, curious, bright-eyed interest in the world around them.

At first, the person might be a bit mystified by these questions and observations because when we're not used to wondering about such things the changes can seem rather subtle.

'I didn't notice anything different!' they say, though the difference seemed clear to me looking in from the outside.

But in time, as we continue to gently explore and I continue to point things out, they begin to notice these things too. They become more sensitive to slight changes and nuances which they'd have missed a short while ago and, without striving, effort or impatience, they begin to catch what's happening more quickly. They begin to see it not once it has happened but *as* it's happening. And finally, they notice it *before* it happens. They come to see that they're *about* to tighten, *about* to hold their breath, *about* to narrow their attention. And, in the process, they also begin to realise that this awareness gives them a choice. Do they let this response unfold, or do they say a quiet no to it? Do they let their breath fix and hold, or do they give it quiet permission to move freely? Do they let their attention narrow and fix or do they say no and remain open and present to themselves and the world around them? Do they try to force their torso into uprightness or will they get out of its way, allowing their spine to move delicately into its own unforced length as they release gently into the welcome support of the ground?

Chapter Twenty-Four
Ease and Movement

It's lovely to be able to find a state of ease, but it's just as important to be able to move and do things in ways that don't disrupt that ease so we can carry it into our activities with us. But as we've seen, many of us habitually move in ways that contradict our body's attempts to manifest ease. Our movements uncentre us. They're unintegrated and uneconomical or overload our muscles with our own body weight causing muscles to spontaneously tighten and brace. So if we want to move with dynamic ease and skilfulness we'll need to make some changes to the ways we coordinate ourselves in activity.

When we think about moving more skilfully it's tempting to think in terms of explicit standards of right and wrong. We want to know what to do based on following some set of procedural instructions: 'Keep a straight back as you lift, move your arm like this, bend your knees,' and so on. We then judge how well we're putting those instructions into practice based on whether it *feels* as if we're doing what we intended. But although this approach seems like common sense it's not as effective as we might think, because explicit instructions are quite limited, and the way a movement feels isn't nearly as helpful a guide as it seems.

The Limits of Instructions

Imagine if someone attempted to give you clear, detailed and easy-to-follow procedural instructions for everything you need to do in your life. We've already seen that there's a place for this type of explicit knowledge. But on its own it's insufficient to enable us to move with real ease and skilfulness.

For a start, relying on sets of instructions limits our possibilities and makes us dependent. It doesn't give us a basis for coming up with lovely new ways of moving when faced with new tasks or unfamiliar situations.

Our bodies and the things we want to do and express with them, and the situations we find ourselves in, are so rich, complex and varied! Even a simple task such as standing up from a chair can be done in numerous ways. We can lean forwards slowly until our weight is over our feet and then straighten our legs. We can lean forwards faster and use the momentum to carry us forwards, straightening our legs as we go. We can walk our pelvis to the edge of the chair on our sitting bones to bring our weight over our feet before standing. We can distribute effort more widely by pushing sensitively with our arms and hands on the arms of the chair as well as with our legs. Any of these ways, and others too, can be skilful and appropriate depending on the circumstances.

Or think about reaching to pick something up from a table. Extending our arms shifts our centre of gravity forwards, which needs to be counterbalanced so we don't fall over. We could do this by leaning very slightly backwards from our ankles as we reach forwards with our arms. Or we could alter the shape and position of our base of support as we reach by putting one foot forward and shifting our weight onto that. Or we could reach out with one arm while raising the other behind us so that its weight counterbalances the one that is reaching forwards. We could even shift onto one leg and—as we reach out with our arm—move the other leg out behind us to counterbalance it.

So even very simple activities like reaching or getting out of a chair present us with many possibilities for how to go about doing them—any of which may be appropriate depending on the circumstances. And the more complex the activity, the more varied and complex these potential choices become.

But the possibilities don't stop with the broad, general patterns of coordination we choose. There's also an infinite variety of *ways* we can carry out each of these general plans. The starting point from which the movement has to unfold is never quite the same. The exact way our limbs are arranged, how our weight is placed, the precise distribution of muscle tone throughout the body and our mood and our emotional state are always a bit different, demanding a fresh response, a slightly different balance of coordination, timing and effort, even for the same action carried out from one time to another. The quality of our attention, the level of emotional and energetic arousal we bring to the task, the timing and speed with which our various body parts move in relationship to each other and the way we use momentum and inertia can all be varied ad-infinitum, affecting the quality, economy and freedom we experience. There is far too much going on, and there are far too many possibilities, for us to be able to reduce skilful movement to explicit, procedural plans.

Feeling as a Guide to Movement

Even if it *were* possible to come up with explicit plans that were sufficiently subtle, flexible and reliable to enable us to find ease and skilfulness in our activities, this would still not be sufficient to ensure we stayed centred, integrated and at ease as we moved. We've seen that our proprioceptive senses can easily become inaccurate and insensitive. But even when they're working at their best they're still not perfect. And even if they were, by the time we notice what they're telling us about the way we're moving, we've already moved and so it's *too late*. If the movement was poorly coordinated, our muscles will already have tightened and braced in response, and whatever ease we started out with will already have been lost. So to move skilfully we're going to need a different yardstick to tell us whether we're on the right track or not.

Pre-Emptive Bracing

Our voluntary actions begin with **intentions**. We form a mental picture of what we're about to do before we do it. Crucially, our body responds to these intentions by getting our system ready *in advance*, activating muscles to provide stabilisation and support for the actions we're about to take *before we've even begun to move*. This means that as soon as you form an intention to move in an unintegrated or uncentred way, or in a way that would overload your muscles with your own body weight, your muscles spontaneously tense up a little to prepare the braced stabilisation and support that will be needed to carry your intention out. It's the same with unhelpful habits. Your system braces to stabilise uncentred, unintegrated habitual movements *before* those movements actually begin.

You can experience some of these **pre-emptive bracing responses** for yourself, right now. If you're sitting down, make ready to stand up from your chair in the way you normally would. I expect that just as you're on the verge of moving there will be a slight tightening and bracing in your body—particularly in your torso and breath—as your system gets ready to stabilise and support you.

If you don't notice any tightening it may be because you've become a little insensitive over the years to this kind of sensory feedback, so here's something that's easier to notice. Try lying down on your back on the floor and then get ready to move into a sitting position by pulling your head and torso straight up off the ground. I'm sure that, just as you're on the verge of moving, you'll be able to feel a pre-emptive bracing in your belly, breath and legs and a tightness in your breathing as your muscles get ready to hold the unsupported weight of your torso and head.

Depending on what we're doing, these pre-emptive bracing responses—which we usually experience most clearly in our torso and breathing—can be quite strong or rather subtle. But they can always be taken as clear little warnings that say 'don't go that way'. They give us a chance to pause, say no, reflect, and make a different, more harmonious choice.

Does any of this sound familiar? We're back in the realm of not-this-not-that. We may not know how to go about the movement in an easy, free, expansive way yet, but we can be sure that it's not like this!

Pre-emptive bracing, then, can act as a channel, gently steering us away from actions that are uncentred and un-integrated, or that overload our muscles, giving us the opportunity to discover fresh new ones which keep us centred as we go, which are integrated, which flow, and which dis-tribute muscular effort widely leaving our system free to continue to manifest dynamic stabilisation even in the midst of activity.

It seems likely to me that pre-emptive bracing helps explain how young children and naturally well-coordinated older people learn to move skilfully without being explicitly taught how or needing to think much about it. When their torso and breathing tightens in response to some unhelpful intention, it feels rather tense and awkward to them so they quite naturally and unselfconsciously don't go that way. Children, in particular, live much more in the moment than most adults. They haven't yet been taught to ignore or override their immediate sense of ease in the pursuit of more abstract goals in the future. They're still sensitive enough to their bodily responses that the pre-emptive tightening which poor movement choices evoke helps to channel them, by a process of elimination, towards ones that are more healthy, open and free. In the next chapter we'll look at how we can develop a practice that will help *us* learn to take advantage of this possibility too.

Chapter Twenty-Five

Exploring Skilful Action

Movement is the song of the body.
—Vanda Scaravelli, Awakening the Spine

Let's say you've decided to put aside a bit of time each day to find out how to take ease into activity and to explore the way you move and do things. How should you go about it?

You'll need to begin this daily practice by choosing an activity to work with. When you're starting out it makes sense for this to be something very simple—perhaps standing up from or sitting down on a chair,[*] reaching out with an arm, bending down to pick something up off the floor, coming onto tiptoes, taking a step or rolling over on the ground. And it also makes sense to begin by working in a slow, gentle way so that you have time to think and don't have to bother about the effects of inertia and momentum which can come into play when you're moving faster.

So let's say you've chosen some simple activity to explore. You may feel an urge to go straight into movement. But rather than rushing in, you will need to pause first and take some time to settle and find a bit of ease in yourself. After all, you can't take ease into movement if you don't have any to begin with.

It's probable, though, that even once you've found some ease, the moment you get ready to go into the activity it will go straight out of the window again! You're likely to get distracted, your focus shifting entirely to what you're about

---

[*] A firm-seated dining chair without arms is ideal for this.

to do rather than staying gently present to your state and where you *are*. Perhaps you'll become subtly anxious about 'getting it right', your breath and musculature tightening with nervous anticipation. Perhaps you'll concentrate and become over-intent about it all. Perhaps you'll lose your connection with the ground, or hold your breath, or otherwise brace in preparation. All your usual habitual doings and interferences will likely get triggered straight away.

But never mind! You spot it happening and gently say no. You put aside your desire to be getting on with the movement, choosing instead to pause and come back to ease, giving it as much time and space as needed. And again, if necessary. And again.

If you notice that you're getting a bit fixed and intent about it all, try moving around freely for a moment. Have a look around you, let your breath go if you've been holding it, and come back to quietness. There's no rush. If this repeated returning to ease is all you end up exploring today, that will be enough.

But let's say that, after a while, you're finding you *can* remain in a quiet state of ease, even in the face of forming the intention to carry out the activity you're working with. Even so, it's likely that just as you're about to go into movement, your torso and breath will pre-emptively brace a little because you were about to move in a habitual way that was unintegrated, or would have uncentred you, or would have been overly effortful, or would have overloaded your muscles with your own body weight.*

It's alright though! This pre-emptive bracing isn't a problem but a helpful *signal*. It's your body letting you

---

* See Chapter Fifteen for a reminder about the sort of things we do that cause spontaneous bracing and interfere with ease in movement.

know that you were asking it to move in a way that it could only carry out by bracing and tightening. How wonderful to have noticed! It gives you a chance to say no to what you were about to do, to pause and come back to quietness and ease, to wonder what it was about the way you were going to move that made your system tense up in preparation, and to think about how you might go about performing the activity in a different way that won't evoke those kinds of bracing responses.

Just as we used the seven qualities to guide our explorations of ease, we can use the four characteristics of skilful action—*integration, centredness, economy* and *flow*—to guide our wonderings and explorations around this. Here are four questions based on them to get you started:

1. Were you going to move in an **integrated** way, allowing many different joints to work harmoniously together? Or would the movement have been fragmented, bracing in one place while moving in another or requiring some of your muscles to bear too much of your own body weight?

   Perhaps there's a different way to coordinate the movement in which everything works together, distributing effort widely throughout your body.

2. Would the way you were going to move have kept you **centred** right through the movement and out the other side? Or would it have *un*centred you, taking your weight towards the edge of your base of support?

   Perhaps there's a way of moving that would enable you to carry out the activity while staying centred as you go.

3. Were you going to move with **economy** or would you have been applying unnecessary effort?

   Perhaps you could think about moving less forcefully. Maybe there are innate movement patterns which could be allowed to unfold and self-organise in their own way, or perhaps this is a situation where you could use gravity or momentum to help you.

4. Is the activity you're exploring made up of a sequence of several smaller movements? Were you giving each of them the time they need and putting them in an order that would have enabled them to **flow** freely from one to another?

   Perhaps it would be better to put some of those smaller movements in a different order or to add some additional steps—maybe shifting your weight from one limb to another, placing your limbs to alter the size or position of your base of support, or pushing or yielding with your limbs to share and distribute effort as you go.

Notice that I'm not telling you what to do or providing explicit instructions for you to follow! There's no formula. Instead we're wondering, exploring and taking time to find out for ourselves. What's *actually* going on here? How might the way we're intending to move be conflicting with our body's natural tendency to manifest ease? Maybe there's a better way. What might it be?

We're not in a hurry, not worried about whether we immediately get it 'right'. It's an experiment, a game. We're bringing an attitude of patience, curiosity and interest to it all.

And so we pause and come back to ease, and having

considered things a little, prepare to move in a way we think might better enable that ease to continue as we carry out the activity.

Perhaps, once again, we notice that our torso and breath pre-emptively tighten as we go to move. So once more we pause, come back to ease, consider, and then try again in another way, taking our time with it, discovering and learning as we go.

Maybe this?

No, my breath tightens a little as I go to move like that.

Or that?

No, not that way either.

Again, if at any point in this process of exploration and discovery you find yourself getting a bit over-intent and fixated on it all, take a break! Breathe out, look around you, move about, maybe take a little walk around the room. Then, when you're ready, gently come back to the activity you've chosen, or perhaps choose a different one to explore for a while.

*Would moving like **this** allow my body to remain free?*

No, it doesn't seem to.

*Or perhaps if I go ever so delicately and freely **this** way . . .*

Ahhh!

Suddenly you find you can go that way freely and easily, the movement unfolding all-of-a-piece as the way you're moving leaves your system free to continue to organise delicious, dynamic stabilisation and grounded support right through the movement and out the other side. It's as if a door that had been locked is suddenly opening, yielding gently to your touch.

We need to stay open and curious in these explorations! Sometimes we'll find that a movement unfolds freely and easily using a coordination that isn't too dissimilar to how we're used to doing it. Perhaps it just takes a shift in balance or timing, or a small change in the particular way we coordinate the movements of our torso, head and limbs. But sometimes we'll find that in order to carry an activity out skilfully, we'll need to coordinate our movements in a very unfamiliar way. Perhaps we'll need to begin with preparatory movements or shifts in position that seem long-winded and unexpected. We may need to find a completely different sequence of movements to the habitual one we're used to using. We may never have moved like this before. The freshness and beauty of a way of moving that reveals itself through this practice may sometimes take us by surprise.

Body Mapping and Movement

We saw earlier that chronic bracing can cause our mental map of our body to become distorted and inaccurate. This can be a particular problem in movement because our intentions are based on this mental map. If the map is inaccurate we'll be asking our body to move in ways that aren't in accord with its actual structure. It will try its best to oblige, but it's unlikely to be able to do so in a well-coordinated, free and easy way.

So as we experiment with movement, it's often helpful to notice whether we're picturing our structure accurately and to gently remind ourselves of how we're *actually* put together. Alexander teachers call this 'body mapping'. For example, you might think:

Here's my head–neck joint, right between my ears.

Are my hips joints really up at the crest of my pelvis where I imagine them? Ah, no, they're here, much lower down.

> *Am I picturing the true extent of my spine, seeing it as the single, strong, flexible structure it is?*
>
> *Am I seeing my arms as the articulated, flexible structures they are?*
>
> *Am I aware of my elbow's potential for movement and that my forearm can rotate as well as bend at the wrist and elbow?*
>
> *Here's the ball-and-socket joint of my shoulder. It's part of my shoulder blade, which can move freely over my ribcage.*
>
> *And here's my collarbone, which connects my shoulder blade and arm to my torso—here, where it meets the breastbone.*

In time, through this practice of gently correcting our mental map of our body, the map becomes more accurate, and as it does so the intentions that are based on it naturally become more in accord with the way things really are.

Beyond the Pause

As we explore these simple but profound things day by day, week by week, observing and learning as we go, our sensitivity and understanding grows. We start to notice preemptive bracing more easily, and find we can say no sooner and more straightforwardly to the unhelpful intentions and habits that led to it. In time, as we circle the problem, we begin to be able to sense intuitively that a particular intention or movement will take us away from ease. And, without becoming rigid or formulaic about it, we start to get a sense of the sort of movements and ways of coordinating ourselves that will *not*. We develop ever more refined procedural and tacit understandings of what is generally helpful and what isn't, and it becomes simpler and easier to find our way into integrated, centred, economical, flowing ways of moving, and to avoid tight, braced, unhelpful ones.

As these abilities become easier and more accessible we become more and more able to apply what we're learning in our everyday lives. Increasingly our old, familiar states of being and the way that we used to move and do things seem awkward and uncomfortable compared to the delicious ease we're discovering in our practice. We catch ourselves distracted, tense, stressed or rushing, and rather than pressing on we take a moment to reset, settle and find some ease. We sense we're about to move in a way that's fragmented, or uncentred, or overly effortful, or sequenced in an unhelpful way, and rather than just following our habit we pause for a moment, find some ease and make a different choice.

In the end, it gets so that often we *don't even need to make the pause first*. We see it all so clearly that finding ease and seeing a way into a harmonious, well-coordinated action happens in the moment, in a heartbeat, in the space between one step and the next, all-of-a-piece.

Perhaps the things I've been talking about in this chapter sound impossibly distant from where you are now. But really it's a very natural process—just a delicate coming back to your true nature. If you give yourself time to reflect and experiment—gently circling the problem, showing up day by day, taking an interest, being willing to consistently be in the process—then gently, bit by bit, you'll discover it for yourself. Remember, we're *designed* to learn and integrate complexity into simplicity. We can *all* do it. We're *integrating animals*. Gradually, in a process beyond words, it happens. You find, to your surprise, that you're able to move and be in the world in a new way.

Chapter Twenty-Six
Using the Floor

So far I've been talking about ease and skill mostly from the perspective of being upright, but it can also be interesting to explore these things while lying on the floor. Just the simple act of stopping what we're doing to lie down quietly for a bit can help bring us out of our habitual busyness, encouraging us to become present and slow down. Being on the floor also takes away the need to balance and find support in the field of gravity, making it feel safer and easier to let go of habitual ways of holding ourselves which may appear to be essential when we're upright.

The Semi-Supine Position

There are numerous positions we can adopt when we lie on the floor.[*] A particular favourite among Alexander teachers is the **semi-supine** position which simply means lying on your back with your knees bent. Most Alexander teachers suggest that people set aside time to lie quietly like this for ten or fifteen minutes every day.

This gentle daily practice can be deceptively powerful. It encourages us to take a break from our busy lives, giving us structured time to quieten, reset and return to balance. The position naturally encourages shortened, braced back muscles to release and lengthen, and increases awareness of our back and spine which gain clear sensory feedback

---

[*] It's best to work on a firm, carpeted floor rather than a softer surface like a couch or bed.

from the firm floor that they don't often receive in the rest of our lives.

When you lie in semi-supine it's important that your head is supported rather than lolling uncomfortably backwards. The traditional advice is to put a book or two under your head so that it's level. You may also want to put a strip of non-slip material under your feet so that you can let go of your legs rather than having to hold on to stop them straightening out under their own weight. Your arms can be by your side, spread out wide, or resting comfortably on your belly.

There's really not much to this semi-supine practice. It's not a difficult thing. Most importantly, you need to *show up*—stop what you're doing at least once a day and actually get on the floor and lie there! For many people, this is the most difficult part. Once you're there, you don't need to be doing anything in particular. All that's needed is a general intention to quieten down, settle and come to ease. If you notice any intentness, concentration, bracing or breath-holding, you can use not-this-not-that to gently explore what it might mean to not be doing those things—to give your torso and breath a chance to move, open and settle in their own time, to give your spine permission to let go into its full, unforced length, and to leave everything else free to find its proper place in its own time and way.

We can get over-intent, busy and effortful about all this, just as we can when we're upright, so we need to take our time and put a bit of gentleness around it, quietly noticing if we're getting busy about not being busy, choosing to make space for our system to settle naturally as it will. If today we're so distracted and uptight that we can't settle, never mind! Remember, it's a *practice* we're engaging in. We don't have to be perfect today. There's no rush. There's always tomorrow. We can trust that in time it will become clearer and easier. Our system will get better at responding to our invitations for it to quieten and settle, and we'll get better at saying no to any inclinations to interfere or unhelpfully hurry it along.

Other Recumbent Positions

Apart from semi-supine, we can adopt many other relaxed positions on the floor. We can be on our front, our back or our side, with our limbs and head organised in all kinds of different ways—straight, curled up, spread out, symmetrical or irregular. Just as when lying semi-supine, we can hold the gentle intention to quieten, settle and find some ease. We can use supportive cushions and beanbags to rest against, lean into or wrap ourselves around. I'd encourage you to take some time each day to investigate some of the possibilities. As you do so, you may find that small—even tiny—shifts in how your head, limbs and torso are placed can enable your structure to receive a little more support from the ground, offering the possibility of ever more delicate release. Over time, these very quiet and gentle explorations can come to feel quite delicious. At the same time they may increase your awareness of subtle sensations associated with holding, and letting go of holding, and this awareness will continue to be available to you as you explore ease and skilfulness when you're upright in the rest of your life.

Music and Regulation

If, despite your best intentions, you find it difficult to quieten and calm down as you lie quietly, it might help to put on some slow, meditative music. Music affects our emotions and nervous system in a very direct way and can be a powerful aid in encouraging our system to quieten down, settle and feel safe—particularly when we're just starting out with the practice. Very calm acoustic or electronic ambient music without a strong beat is a good choice. Even when we've been doing the work for a long time this can continue to be useful, bringing us back to calmness and balance if we're going through a stressful time in our lives, or even if we've just had a difficult day.

Exploring Movement on the Floor

As we begin to be able to access a neutral, easy state on the floor, we can begin to explore movement there, too. Many of the movements we can make on the floor are less practised and habitual than the everyday things we do when we're upright. The habits around them tend to be less strong and ingrained making it relatively easy to make different choices.

Working with movement on the floor is also helpful because the pre-emptive bracing that precedes uncentred, unintegrated movements is often stronger and more noticeable when we're horizontal than when we're upright. We may not yet have developed the sensitivity to notice the more delicate pre-emptive tightening sensations that precede many of our upright actions. But suppose we're lying down and carelessly go to lift an extended arm or leg off the ground from the shoulder or hip joint, or to roll over clumsily. The horizontal weight of our limbs, torso and head will put our musculature under a lot of strain. We'll almost certainly be able to sense the warning tightening and holding in our torso and breathing that accompanies it. This makes working on the floor particularly helpful when we're starting out with the practice.

There are so many interesting ways to move on the floor—from large, expansive gestures and shifts in position to tiny, exquisite micro-movements. We can move our arms, legs and head, folding and unfolding our limbs, either in contact with the floor or raised above it. We can roll over onto our backs, sides or fronts in numerous ways. We can roll right across the room if we want to. We can use gravity to help us—shifting our arms or legs across us or lifting them from the floor, taking advantage of their weight to help our heavy torso and head to roll over without excess effort. We can stretch and bend, actively using our limbs to support and enable further movements—lifting, placing, pushing and yielding with our hands, feet, elbows and knees, using skilful limb placement to distribute muscular effort when rolling or raising our head, torso or limbs from the floor. And, in time, we can begin to explore movement on all fours, stretching, curling, and shifting our weight to take cat-like steps with our hands and feet.

Chapter Twenty-Seven
Towards Complexity

So far I've introduced some principles and practices that, when explored regularly, can help nudge your system towards a state of dynamic freedom and ease and allow you to take that ease skilfully into activity. I've been talking mostly with regard to very simple activities—standing up from a chair or sitting down, reaching and bending, shifting weight and taking a step, crawling, rolling over and so on. We can go a long way just by working with these simple movements. But really they're only building blocks. Sooner or later, if we're going to do anything useful or interesting with them, we will have to combine them, joining them together into increasingly complex sequences (putting them one after the other) and combinations (making different movements at the same time).

Practical versus Exploratory Sequences

Combinations and sequences can serve pragmatic, practical purposes, such as in the reaching, grasping, spiralling, retracting and placing movements that we might do while washing up, or the rolling, placing and pushing of limbs needed to come onto all fours or to move into a squat and up into standing when we're getting up from a bed or the floor. But as we began to see at the end of the last chapter, we can also work in more open-ended, exploratory ways, improvising combinations and sequences which are not aimed towards any practical end but simply at exploring ourselves in action, finding new ways to move by being curious and following our mood and interest—squatting and standing, lunging, changing our base of support, shifting our weight, turning, spiralling, balancing, taking steps of varying lengths in different directions, moving our arms, our shoulders and our head, going down to the floor and up again, all the time discovering more about ourselves and our bodies and how they like to move and function.

Initially it's best to play with sequences slowly, taking time to discover how delicately we can move, how refined, free and open we can be, how movement can blend and lead into movement, and where this can take us. This kind of open exploration can come to feel quite delicious, and the better we get at saying no to habits and responses that don't align with freedom and ease, the more delicious it becomes.

Letting Go of the Pause

When we were looking at very simple movements we practised pausing before moving, taking time to find ease so that we could take that ease into the movement with us. To begin with, as we experiment with longer sequences of movements, it's helpful to continue to work this way, pausing to find ease between each step of the sequence before moving on to the next from that clear, open place. It's a calm, deliberate practice that depends on moving slowly enough for momentum not to come into play, allowing us to pause as and when we need to.

In time, though, you'll find that you no longer need to pause before each step of the sequence. You will *already* be present and breathing, free and open in your musculature, and in dynamic stabilisation and grounded support, because those qualities will not have been lost in the previous step—you will have kept them with you right through the movement and out the other side. And even if ease is momentarily lost, you will no longer need to stop and pause to regain it—you can find it again in the moment, as you go. At the same time you will be becoming more sensitive to the sorts of movements that interfere with ease, and more adept at channelling your actions away from them towards ones that do not. More and more you'll find that you can move easily and freely from movement to movement while staying open and free, without pausing, each step blending smoothly, imperceptibly into the next until it all becomes a single, unfolding flow of action.

Speeding Up

As we begin to find it easier to allow our system to remain in a state of dynamic ease and flow in activity, we can begin exploring faster movements in which momentum and inertia come into play. Doing this, we will find that at times we need to lean in to or away from our direction of travel as we speed up or slow down, taking account of the apparent momentary shifts in the direction of gravity that momentum and inertia induce.[*] Fortunately this is easy to grasp intuitively. It's not difficult to do. We all have an innate understanding of how it works.

As we move faster, we find that often we *can't* pause and consider in the middle of a sequence of movements anymore even if we wanted to, because if we try to stop our momentum will carry us onwards. Instead we can begin to explore allowing movements to continue under their own momentum while we use that space to direct their course, find some ease, and be ready for the next ones.

---

[*] You can refer back to page 61 for more information about this.

Sometimes, when we're exploring longer, faster sequences, we find we can be at ease for a short time but soon get behind or ahead of ourselves, becoming overwhelmed so that we brace and seize up. We can work with this by chunking—moving fast through a short part of a sequence (as much as we can do without bracing) then stopping, coming to neutral, breathing, giving ourselves as much time as needed to find ease before going into another short burst and so on. After a while we find we need to stop for shorter and shorter periods; it takes less and less time to reset between each chunk until everything begins to join up, and we find we can make increasingly long, fast sequences of movements while staying easy, open and free right the way through.

Movement and Music

Music can be a powerful aid to playing with movement in the exploratory ways I've been describing in this chapter. Its rhythm and emotional content originate in the integrated movements that musicians need to use if they're to play or sing well. Part of the magic of music is that we can absorb a sense of this just through listening. The sounds can nudge us towards integrated ways of moving that we might not stumble across so easily on our own.

If you start exploring things this way, it makes sense to begin with very slow, meditative sounds. The floor is a good place to start. As you lie there, let the music gently seep into your awareness allowing it to affect you and seeing what impulses arise in response. Maybe large, expansive movements will be evoked, but it could also be tiny, delicate ones. In time, you can come gradually to your feet, moving meditatively on all fours or standing. Ultimately, you can speed things up, choosing more vigorous music to explore faster movements and a wider range of expression.

Skilled Pastimes

As we become more adept at finding ease and skilfulness, we can bring those qualities to ever-expanding areas of our lives—to our daily chores, our work and our relationships—making everything easier. In time, it's likely that you'll also want to bring your increasing skilfulness to any artistic or athletic activities you take part in. So many activities can benefit from this! Music, drama, dancing, singing, running, horse riding, swimming, archery, tai chi, yoga and meditation to name a few. People are often surprised and delighted to find how their performance and enjoyment in these activities increase as they approach them with an emphasis on ease, presence and freedom rather than focusing excessively on the end result. At the same time, the challenges such activities present, and the focused practice they demand, give us one of the best ways to broaden and deepen our understanding of ease and skilfulness more generally.

Every skilled pastime has different schools of thought on how to go about learning it. People sometimes have very entrenched views about these different ways, and inevitably some of them will be a better fit for our principles of ease and skill than others. It's not going to be helpful to approach swimming, playing a musical instrument or horse riding through a teaching method that emphasises muscular holding, control or rigidity. A teacher who emphasises relaxed freedom in the activity is likely to be a much better fit. We need to find someone whose teaching encourages awareness, openness, flow and economy of movement, and who is as concerned with helping us take care of ourselves in the activity as they are with competitiveness and outward achievement.

Many Alexander teachers specialise in working in specific artistic and sporting fields, bringing a specialist knowledge along with their general knowledge of how to access ease and skill in activity. Finding one of these would be an excellent place to start. Otherwise, take some time to visit several teachers and choose one whose approach seems compatible with what you're beginning to experience through your practice.

If you're a beginner you're in an ideal position because you have a clean slate. Right from the start you can be working in ways that will support you in finding ease as your ability grows. If you've already been involved with the activity for a long time, though—and particularly if you've been under the influence of a more rigid, controlled approach—you may need to begin with a period of *unlearning* as you realise that habits you've got into (some of which you might have become quite attached to) are not helping you. You might have to agree with yourself to allow some time to go backwards, putting in place more beneficial foundations before going forwards again.

Chapter Twenty-Eight
Energetic Release

Earlier in the book we saw that when someone has had experiences where expressing their emotional responses had negative social consequences, they may suppress or repress those feelings, keeping them locked up inside with muscular tension. Over time, this can contribute to chronic tension and bracing in their body, and reduce their ability to feel and express their emotions. When we've been suppressing or repressing emotions with muscular tension and begin to let that tension go through a practice like the Alexander Technique, we may find that we go through a period—or several periods—when those emotions start to surface and work their way out. This may be completely unexpected. Either in a lesson or just going about our lives, we're suddenly overcome by waves of anger or sadness that don't seem to have an obvious, proportionate cause in the present. Sometimes these feelings will be accompanied by memories of the original events connected to the feelings. But they can also be free-floating, leaving us unsure where the feelings come from. What's usually important, though, is not identifying the underlying cause so much as the fact that these old feelings and muscular tensions are finally letting go.

Some people don't mind feelings and memories from the past coming up: others find it uncomfortable. Fortunately, Alexander work tends to be quite gentle with repressed feelings. It's usually not like pulling a cork out of a champagne bottle but more like gently letting out air from a balloon. Having said that, a few people may have experienced a degree of distress or trauma in the past that means they may need additional help from a counsellor or therapist to support them and help them make sense of things while this process of release is going on.

Discharging Survival Energy

One form of emotional release that sometimes occurs in Alexander lessons can be thought of as a discharge of unused survival energy. Survival energy is the 'charge' aroused in us for self-defence or flight when we're anxious or frightened. Once the situation that gave rise to this charge is over, the energy that was aroused needs to dissipate or it will remain locked up in our system. The muscle tone that was mobilised for fight or flight needs to let go, the hormones and other chemicals that were pumped into the bloodstream to prepare the body to defend itself need to be discharged or reabsorbed, and blood flow needs to be redirected from the muscles back to other organs in the body.

The body has various mechanisms which are designed to help with this process of discharge. We may spontaneously shake, yawn, stretch, sigh, shudder, sob or laugh. Tears may help clear chemicals and hormones associated with the heightened feelings, and we may experience heat, cold or tingling as blood flow is redirected away from the muscles. Similar responses can be observed in other animals. When a wild animal has had a narrow escape, such as a brush with a predator, it will often spontaneously shiver, shake or rush about once the danger has passed to release any unused survival energy, allowing its system to shift back towards an easy, open state.

When a person carrying unresolved survival energy comes for Alexander lessons, they may find that at one time or another they start shaking, or experiencing other symptoms of energetic discharge such as pins and needles or sensations of hot and cold as muscular bracing that has been holding back the resolution of survival energy from the past releases. This is generally nothing to worry about—just a natural, much-needed resetting of the system.

We'll be looking further at various emotional aspects of the work in the remainder of the book.

Part Five
Deepening The Practice

Chapter Twenty-Nine
Contact, Attunement and Expression

The body says what words cannot.
—Martha Graham, atrib.

Although so far we've been thinking quite deeply about ease and skill, from another perspective we've also been looking at them in a rather limited way because we've generally only considered ourselves in isolation without giving much thought to the need to be in relationship with other people and objects. But in real life, we're in constant, ever-changing relationship with the people and things around us and with the thoughts and feelings they evoke. In this chapter we're going to begin thinking about this, and particularly about how we make **contact** and **attune** to people and things, and how we **express** ourselves through our bodies and voices.

Contact

To be in relationship with people and objects we first need to come into contact with them in some way, either psychologically or physically. When our neuromuscular system is dynamically stabilising and supporting us, we have the opportunity for that to be a living, sensitive and responsive contact.

When you're asleep, your body is *literally* in contact with the sheets and mattress but that's not the kind of contact I mean. Or if you collapse in front of the television at the end of the day, your body is *literally* in contact with the sofa, but that's not the sort of contact I mean either, because there's no alive, physical, emotional or mental connection with the thing you're in contact with.

Similarly, if someone you don't like were to come up to you and give you an unwelcome hug, you'd most likely stiffen and tense up. Even if you decided to put up with it and play along, mentally and physically you'd be recoiling and seeking to disconnect. Though there would be literal physical contact between you, this wouldn't be the sort of contact I'm talking about either.

The sort of contact I mean is a dynamic, responsive, *alive* contact, in which we meet others and objects in the world around us clearly and intentionally. We're neither collapsing and detaching nor pushing the person or thing away. We're right there with them.

Imagine being a skilled violinist and the quality with which you'd hold the instrument as you played. You wouldn't grasp the neck roughly and insensitively, and neither would you let it just lie there like a dead thing in the crook of your hand. More likely, you'd bring a delicate, live presence and warmth to the contact, perhaps as you might if you were holding a young child's hand. Or imagine sitting quietly and easily opposite someone you are very fond of and reaching out to take their hands in yours. Hopefully there'd be an alive, connected softness about the contact which would help you to connect with them with presence and gentleness. Even a simple task like washing the dishes can involve a kind of sensitive, present, dynamic contact as we hold, lift, wipe and place down the plates and cutlery. It's certainly more enjoyable that way.

Our ability to make this kind of contact is influenced

by the degree to which our system is able to organise dynamic stabilisation and support. The responsiveness of dynamic organisation, together with the presence and open attention that accompanies it, helps bring us into a living physical, mental and emotional contact with the person or thing.

Sometimes it's difficult to make contact like this. This may be partly to do with the habits of holding, bracing, concentration and mental disconnection that we've talked about already. But there may also be barriers specific to contact with other people which have a basis in emotional wounds from the past—particularly if those wounds happened when we were very young. For some, contact with others may have come to feel threatening and unsafe causing their system to go into fear-based defensive reactions, tightening, withdrawing or freezing, making an alive, responsive contact impossible.

It can be interesting to bring exploring contact into your practice. You can begin with objects—leaning gently against a wall or gently holding some delicate object, discovering what it's like to maintain a sense of ease, lightness and flexibility in that contact and in yourself as a whole, breathing lightly, freely and easily as you do so.

In time, you can begin to explore contact with willing friends, teachers or co-students—meeting hand to hand or back to back, leaning shoulder to shoulder or doing whatever else feels comfortable to explore together, observing how you respond. Do you become subtly or obviously anxious? Do you collapse a little bit, losing a sense of yourself? Or perhaps you become a little rigid and fixed, or try too hard so that concentration and effort gets in the way of a simple, clear connection.

Perhaps, though, through growing awareness and practising not-this-not-that (wondering what we *don't* want, what's *not* it, what we're up to that's interfering with it) we gradually discover a new quality of contact. We find we can let go of held, braced or collapsed ways of connecting and calm and settle our system enough to trust a little, finding that it's safe to quietly be with one another in a more clear and open way.

Attunement

It's wonderful to make contact, but we also need to be able to *maintain* contact with people and things that are moving or responding to us, attuning to the shifting forces and energies that we meet from moment to moment.

Think about standing on a moving bus or train. As it shifts beneath us we must make corresponding movements to remain upright. If we're holding on with an arm, it will need to continuously adjust to the roll and sway while the grip of our fingers adjusts to take account of the irregular motion. We might accommodate ourselves to the movement in a rather awkward, braced way—maybe even having to catch ourselves now and again before we fall if we fail to accurately anticipate what's needed. But ideally we'll be sensitively attuned to the vehicle's movement, moving in sympathy, sensing just the right shifts and adjustments needed to stay relaxedly upright even as it moves beneath us.

In a similar way, a musician needs to be in harmony with their instrument and how it's responding to their touch. A violinist has to be sensitive to the sound they produce as they draw their bow across the string, modulating the force and speed 'just so' to produce the tone and phrasing they're after, consistently and sensitively responding to what they hear.

Most important of all is the ability to attune to other people, enabling us to connect and synchronise emotionally with each other in close relationships, to communicate our state and our feelings at a non-verbal level, and to take part in skilful activities such as dancing, music-making and all kinds of physical closeness and intimacy.

As with contact, our ability to attune benefits from the sensory sensitivity and responsiveness that goes along with dynamic stabilisation and support. The degree to which we can attune to others is related to the extent to which we can find ease and move skilfully while staying close and energetically open to another. Imagine, as we did in Chapter Six, that you're standing opposite a friend with your hands meeting theirs palm to palm. If they were to slowly move their hands around and you were to follow that movement accurately and precisely so as to stay in full, sensitive contact with them, the ongoing adjustment would need to be not only with the joints of your hands, fingers and arms but with *all* of you—an integrated response that allowed your centre of gravity and base of support to shift as needed to keep you centred and free, enabling the dynamic sensitivity and responsiveness of the contact to continue as you moved and breathed together.

It's lovely when we're able to be in tune with and respond to each other in this way, having an intuitive sense of where the other person is and where they're going while they are able to sense and respond to us in turn, the mutual attunement allowing us to enter states where aspects of ourselves that are beyond words can be shared.

Once again, we can explore these things in our practice

with a willing friend, partner, teacher or co-student, meeting hand to hand, or back to back, or side to side, or in any other way that feels right, and then taking that contact into movement, staying in sensitive touch as we wordlessly negotiate how to move together. We may find it good to do this to music, allowing the sounds to inspire new movements, and new ways of feeling, sensing and being with and responding to each other.

Exploring like this can teach us lots about ourselves. We may notice that at certain times (or even all the time) we push the other person rigidly away as if to protect ourselves from them, or excessively give in, collapsing a little, or becoming overwhelmed in the face of real or imagined pressure from the other. Or we may become a little frozen and rigid preventing an easy interplay and exchange with the other person, or withdraw slightly from the situation through mental disconnection or dissociation.

Sometimes we may notice that these ways of responding to our partner bear some similarities to the ways we tend to be in relationships generally, so this practice can also help us discover things about our relational patterns and boundaries. As we explore we may begin to understand better where our edges are—what it feels like to healthily compromise or to hold our ground, where we're willing to let others in and where we're not. Taking it in turns to lead or to yield we find that each end of that continuum needs to contain a bit of the other. We must be able to keep a sense of ourselves even as we yield, and of sensitivity to the other even when we take the lead. We discover both our power and the ability to relinquish it appropriately if we choose. We find we can merge with another for a while if we wish and return to ourselves when we need to. And, in time, we may find that some of these learnings start to manifest naturally in our everyday lives as well.

Expression

We've seen that some of our actions are aimed at getting practical stuff done (getting up from a chair, reaching out to pick something up, doing the dishes, walking from A to B), while others are directed towards exploring and enjoying movement for its own sake or for fostering contact and connection. But we can also use our actions to *express* things, moving or making sounds to show our feelings and emotions to ourselves and others.

As well as being felt inside of us, emotions tend to be expressed through our bodies by the shapes we adopt and the movements we make. When we're happy, we smile: when we're sad, we frown. We shrink away from things that repel, disgust or frighten us and lean in towards things we like or are excited by. If we feel alive and vibrant our face, shoulders and chest open and relax, whereas if we feel sad and hopeless our head falls and our shoulders and thorax may tend to collapse into an unhappy slump—or we might cry, our shoulders moving rhythmically with each sob. We may gesticulate in joy or sadness, and dance, sing or play a musical instrument to express an infinite variety of feelings.

This relationship between our emotions and the postures, shapes, movements and gestures that reflect them runs deep. It's difficult to feel an emotion without some corresponding subtle or obvious expressive shift in our body, even if we try to cover it up.

Emotional expression can be spontaneous or voluntary. Sometimes something happens and our feelings about it immediately express through the body. We smile, laugh or recoil without thinking about it at all. But we can also *deliberately* express a feeling through consciously making movements to show on the outside what's being thought and felt on the inside, or to evoke or intensify feelings we wish to show others or experience for ourselves. Getting up in the morning and opening the curtains to find a sunny day outside, we may exaggerate the spreading movement of our arms, helping us to express our delight and to revel in just how lovely it is. Or in telling our partner about our bad day, we may exaggerate our sagging shoulders and the physical heaviness that goes with the feeling to gain a bit of sympathy or to bring home to ourselves what a rotten time we're having.

Many of us, however, have become a little stilted in our ability to express. We may have received all sorts of messages that warn against the open expression of feelings. We may have learned to value reasoned, controlled movements and actions and vocalisations over free, expansive, expressive ones. For some of us, the injunction against feeling and expressing may have been so strong that just the *thought* of expressing ourselves freely, or of being seen to do so, can bring up feelings of fear, shame and avoidance, leading to bracing and awkwardness.

Our practice can help us become aware of ways we block and stifle the urge to express ourselves as it arises within us. A simple way to explore this is to take a bit of time to quieten down and put our body in charge, really listening for how it wants to move and giving it permission to do so. When we're not imposing our more everyday, goal-driven desires onto our bodies, and if we are open to the possibility, we often find some unexpected emotional impulse arises—perhaps to move our torso, our head, our limbs, our hands or our feet, or to make some gesture or some sound with our voice. Something within us wants to move and be seen or heard. Maybe it's a part of us that's been repressed, or which compulsive busyness and distraction have not allowed to surface so far. Can we give it a bit of space now? Perhaps there will be some impetus to rock, sway, gesture, bend, curl or step. Perhaps we'll find an urge to sing, hum, sigh, yell or make some other sound that's within us waiting for a chance to come out.

As we explore like this, we may find that habitual ways of moving and responding get in the way, taking us out of the moment and the feeling. Or we may feel safer and more in control if we're trying at some level to 'get it right'—over-controlling and second-guessing what our body wants to do. Or we may notice tightening or resistance arising in our body born of fear or shame about making ourselves and our inner world visible in this way. Even if we're doing the exercise on our own we may feel very awkward about it.

Perhaps, though, with practice and patience, we can notice these interfering responses and blocks as they arise and very gently say no to them. Once again we can use not-this-not-that—but this time with a focus on saying no to habits and responses that get in the way of freely expressing our feelings and emotions. Rather than tightening, or avoiding the feelings, we take the risk of staying open and allowing them to reveal themselves. In time we may find that quietly allowing this kind of free expressive movement or sound can bring up surprisingly strong feelings in us that have previously been hidden or denied.

The urge to express through movement and sound is

closely tied to music and dancing, and these are some of the best ways to take these explorations further. Try putting on some music and see what movements it suggests to you. See if you can go with them. The power of music to catch us emotionally can put us in touch with previously unexplored parts of ourselves and encourage us into new, unfamiliar feelings associated with them. We may find that there are many more ways to move and use our bodies to feel and express than we've been allowing ourselves.

If you already like dancing, this kind of exploration may be a pleasure from the start. If you're not used to it, though, you may encounter quite strong resistance in yourself. All sorts of internal judgement and shame can come up. But by staying with the process, using not-this-not-that, gently saying no to tightenings and blocks that get in the way, you may in time find a loosening and softening in yourself.

Sometimes we shy away from certain styles of music because they bring up feelings that we find uncomfortable or don't want to acknowledge in ourselves, so it can be interesting to try moving to music you wouldn't normally listen to. You might even consider joining a conscious dance or contact improvisation class. Moving expressively with others, and being seen as you do so, can feel challenging. Even if you usually feel comfortable dancing with others you may, as your practice deepens, notice new resistances and deeper layers of interference getting in the way of allowing expressive movement to flow freely through you.

Staying patiently with any emotional discomfort these practices bring up can, over time, help you access and express feelings more easily in your everyday life and relationships with others, too. Feeling, expressing and processing emotions becomes easier. You may find that muscular bracing in the area around your heart, shoulders and belly naturally begins to release and open, enabling more unselfconscious expression of feelings of warmth, love, enthusiasm and connection. As the muscles of your mouth, throat, jaw, vocal cords and breath become less held and more able to respond freely to your impulses to communicate, your voice becomes lighter, freer and more flexible. You find you can laugh, sing and speak more freely, and if you feel difficult emotions you're more able to express them clearly and appropriately, and let them go when they've run their course rather than getting stuck in them.

Artistic Expression

The most refined way to consciously express feelings through the body is perhaps found in formal performance arts such as acting, music and dancing. These can be some of the most challenging activities we can undertake, requiring us to make complex, technically demanding movements (physically playing the right notes, speaking the right lines, dancing the correct steps) which also express authentic emotion so that these complementary aspects of the performance come together in harmony.

Our Alexander practice can be a great resource in these endeavours, helping us to find ways of coordinating ourselves that meet the activity's technical demands while simultaneously expressing the emotional content, keeping us in the healthy, free, easy and dynamic state that is conducive to performing at our best.

Once again, we can approach this through not-this-not-that. We can stay clear about the technical demands of the performance while allowing ourselves to feel the emotions, saying no to responses that arise in us which take us away from *either*. In time, we may find that we begin to discover ways of being and moving that integrate all aspects of the performance into a living, breathing whole. Discovering how to bring this about for ourselves can be one of the most interesting, enriching and worthwhile experiences we can have.

Chapter Thirty
Trauma

I've often been struck by the extent to which some people find it fairly straightforward to access a little more ease and skilfulness in themselves, while for others change happens frustratingly slowly. Often the difficulty is due to underlying emotional factors. Sometimes the cause lies in our very early development. Certain experiences in our first few months and years can lead to deeply embedded emotional responses, ways of viewing the world, and patterns of muscular tension or collapse which can get in the way of our most earnest desire to change.

Another source of the trouble may be difficult experiences we've had at any point in our lives that have become locked into our system through trauma. These can leave us prone to chronically over- or under-aroused, anxious states which make accessing ease much more difficult than it would otherwise be. In this chapter we're going to look at this kind of deeply embedded anxiety before going on, in the following one, to look at some common early emotional patterns that can get in the way of ease, and to think about how we might gently shift them.

Causes of Trauma

For some or us, anxiety doesn't run too deep. It's picked up from everyday pressures and expectations, and it doesn't take us long to calm down again if we decide that's what we want to do. For others, though, it may have deeper, more traumatic roots.

Trauma can be very deep or relatively mild. It occurs when we have experiences which are so overwhelming that our brain is unable to process and make sense of them as they're happening. It can occur when we're very young, arising from certain types of interactions with our carers, in which case it can have a significant impact on our subsequent development and is known as **developmental trauma**. It can also happen later in life due to overwhelmingly frightening or difficult events, or it can build up over longer periods of time due to chronic assaults on our dignity and sense of self such as are experienced if we feel trapped in circumstances in which we feel powerless, disrespected or controlled.

Usually the various aspects of an event—the things we see, sense, think and feel while it's going on—are integrated by our brain into a single picture so that they can be made sense of, understood, put in the past and filed away as a normal memory. However, if our brain is overwhelmed during the experience, this process may not complete as it should. Instead, the different parts of the experience remain fragmented. They're not processed, integrated and filed away as being finished but remain in our system as if the situation were still going on.

Whenever something happens in the present that reminds us of the original traumatic experience (perhaps seeing a car like the one in the crash or meeting someone who reminds us of the person who tormented us), these fragments can get reactivated causing our body to respond as if the original event were happening right now. We may get flooded with anxiety and other negative emotions which are out of proportion to the current situation. We may experience 'flashbacks'—intrusive memories of those events which can include the replaying of sensory experiences we had at the time (body memories). The physical manifestations of these strong emotional responses may include sensory disturbances such as shaking, pins and needles or feelings of hot and cold. In some cases, these responses can be strong enough to feel frightening or overwhelming in themselves, causing us to push them away or close them down with muscular tension, preventing them from resolving and contributing to the experience remaining locked in our system.

Trauma may also lead to experiences of immobilisation in which we find it difficult to take action, or of dissociation, in which a person feels detached from their body and their surroundings as if looking in on themselves from the outside. These responses are linked to the freeze and flop parts of our primitive defensive mechanism and can make it particularly difficult to deal with the demands of everyday life.

Resolving Trauma

Whether trauma is debilitating or relatively mild, resolving it generally requires two things. First we need to learn how to regulate our anxiety responses so that we're not thrown into a dysregulated state whenever the traumatic material is triggered. There are some suggestions for regulating and calming your nervous system in Appendix C which may help with this. Once we can do this we may want to allow the traumatic memories into awareness slowly and gently enough that they don't overwhelm us. This gives our brain the chance to integrate and make sense of them so that it can then file them away in the past as normal memories. This gentle process of integration is called titration, and to begin with it may require specialised help from a therapist.

When trauma is relatively mild, Alexander Technique lessons with a trauma-aware teacher may in themselves be sufficient to resolve it. Over time, the calming effect of the lessons and practice, together with the ongoing gentle, regulating hands-on contact from the teacher, may encourage the trauma to integrate and settle in its own way.

If the trauma is more serious, effective trauma therapy is increasingly available. In addition, increasing numbers of Alexander teachers are trained and experienced in working directly with trauma. If you find such a teacher, it may be possible to safely process any deeper trauma that comes up in the course of your lessons.

Chapter Thirty-One
Emotional Blocks

All of us carry at least a few wounds and adaptions from our very early years because the world we're born into, and the pressures it puts individuals and families under, are so far from what our nervous system evolved to expect. These adaptions may form fairly untroublesome parts of our personality. But if we needed to adapt to more difficult situations in more extreme ways, the muscular tension and developmental trauma this can cause will have significant impacts on our ability to access ease and skilfulness in our lives later on.

In seeking to understand these early adaptions and wounds I've been particularly drawn to Wilhelm Reich (1897–1957) and those who have built on his work. Reich noticed that babies and young children tend to adapt to pressures and difficulties in their relationships with their carers in more or less predictable ways at different stages of their development, and that particular patterns of muscular holding or collapse tend to accompany these ways of adapting. Reich called these patterns 'character structures'. His model of them was based on his understanding of the inextricable relationship between mind, body, and emotions which makes it a good fit for the Alexander Technique.

His work suggests that our early history can leave us with difficulties in particular areas of human experience.

The most relevant of these for our purposes are:*

- Difficulties with feeling **safe** and being **present**.
- Difficulties around dealing with our **wants and needs**.
- Difficulties in our ability to **trust** and **express** ourselves.
- Difficulties with being able to **release** and **let go**.

Whether we feel we've been deeply negatively affected by our past experiences, or believe that we're actually rather well adjusted, it's worth considering if any of these patterns apply to us, even if only a little, and whether they sometimes get in the way of our ability to access greater skilfulness and ease. Let's look at them more deeply.

Difficulties With Presence and Safety

When we are very young, in the months just before and after we are born, our senses are the centre of our existence. Without language, concepts and mental models there isn't even a clear sense of separation between ourselves and the world around us. There is touch, light, dark, colour, sound, taste, pleasure, pain, fear and the internal sensations of the body—and particularly of the breath, always moving.

In this state, we're at the mercy of forces outside our control, helpless in the face of other people's actions and our body's spontaneous responses. If our nervous system senses dangers such as falling, frightening sounds, or the threat of being abandoned (which means death to a young

---

* While there is broad agreement about the nature of the different character structures, there is no generally agreed terminology for them. Reich's own labelling, in particular, is often rejected as being outdated and pathologising. The approach I'm using here is most influenced by Laurence Heller and Tim Brown's work. (There are two further character structures which I haven't included. These develop a bit later, and are less straightforwardly relatable to an Alexander Technique context.)

child), fear sweeps through us which we cannot calm on our own. If we're hurt, hungry or cold, pain arises with no ability to self-soothe or any understanding of a future time when the pain will end. Our only refuge lies in dependable others who have the understanding to not only keep us safe, but to keep us *feeling* safe.

As humans, we're born with the expectation that we'll find this kind of supportive care waiting for us when we come into the world. We arrive with our eyes wide, searching for the friendly, welcoming eyes of another. When our gaze is met with the loving gaze of our carers, our nervous system registers safety. We relax, sensing that we're secure and won't be abandoned.

From such a place, where we are held, nurtured, soothed and kept safe, our attention can wander freely, moving from thing to thing, from sensation to sensation, without needing to shy away through fear or excessive discomfort. We discover what it means to just *be*—to be present to the world and to our experience without agenda or self-protectiveness.

Within that open awareness are the continuous movements of the breath. Without the constant distractions of thought, and the busyness that comes when we're older, these sensations are at the heart of our experience of ourselves. When their continuous coming and going is first experienced in the context of warmth and safety it becomes a *resource* for the rest of our life—a place we can go to whenever we need to feel safe and secure. Its presence gives us, at the most basic level, confirmation that we're here—that we *exist*.

Throughout these early months we begin to discover our edges. Through interacting with our carers we start to learn where our body ends and other people and the rest of the world begin. And through exploring ourself and our physicality through movement, touch and vision we begin to gain a sense of our capabilities and of our physical form. We starts to possess our own body.

These things—a sense of safety and belonging, the accompanying freedom in our musculature, free awareness, free breath, and a sense of the boundaries and structure of our physical form—are at the centre of our developing sense of ourselves as healthy, differentiated beings.

If things *don't* go so well, however—if we're *not* safely met and held—our experience may be very different. Instead of a feeling that the world and other people are generally safe, we may be left with a core feeling of danger and uncertainty. We may fail to gain a true sense of our physical boundaries and edges and be left feeling rather amorphous and scattered. It may be difficult to feel fully present and 'here'. This lack of presence and safety may, in turn, make it difficult for us to connect to others. And rather than being experienced as a positive resource, the sensations of breathing may tend to make us feel insecure, or even panicky, when they come into awareness.

If this has been your experience it can make exploring the Alexander Technique more of a challenge. If the pattern isn't too deep, things may settle and resolve just through the lessons if the teacher is willing to be very gentle and patient, and you are willing to give it the time and space it needs. The calming things you're learning, and the gentle, non-invasive touch that is experienced with a trauma-aware teacher can be invaluable, calming your nervous system, helping you establish safety and a sense of your physical edges and boundaries, and allowing you to connect safely with your breath.

For some people, though, even this may be too much. Lessons may be experienced as overwhelming or simply not be beneficial due to these underlying factors getting in the way. If this is the case, more specialised help such as craniosacral work or body psychotherapy may be more helpful to begin with.

Difficulties Around Wants and Needs

Hopefully when we're very young we'll get enough of what we need. We'll get enough food and warmth and enough care, and attention. When this is not the case, however, we can end up with a core feeling of unfulfilled longing— a sense of *lack* that can deeply affect how we are in the world and our relationships with others. This can manifest in several ways. On the one hand, we might *identify* with that feeling of lack, having a constant sense of victimhood and being hard done by. We may be chronically unsatisfied, with a heavy, collapsed air about us, coupled with a similarly heavy, collapsed quality in our body. This can express partly as a loss of ability to be in sensitive contact with the ground. We may come to rest heavily on the Earth beneath us rather than being in the sort of dynamic relationship with it that allows grounded support to activate. Psychologically we may tend towards low mood or depression and always be hoping that others will take care of us.

An alternative outcome might be that we unconsciously reject the feeling of unfulfilled longing and refuse to identify with it. We may decide instead that we have *no* needs, taking on a persona of rugged independence. This may feel more powerful, but it still leaves us isolated while our needs remain unacknowledged.

Finally, we may project our unfulfilled needs outwards,

becoming a compulsive helper, trying to assuage our sense of need where we see it reflected in those around us. We may always be exhausting ourselves helping others—often while feeling resentful about the perceived ingratitude of those same others and about our own still unmet needs. We may carry a firmly set jaw and a heavy presence as we clump around virtuously taking care of everyone but ourselves.

Any of these patterns can interfere with learning a practice like the Alexander Technique. If we have taken the first route it can be hard to raise the energy to commit to learning and change. Everything is hopeless anyway, so why bother trying? We may experience our body primarily as a place of discomfort, lack and suffering and shy away from paying it attention and being kind to it.

If we've decided, on the other hand, that we have no needs, then there's no incentive to try to meet them. And if we have adopted the role of helper it might feel strange, selfish or wrong to put so much thought and interest into ourselves. In any case, doing so would mean admitting to ourselves that we *have* needs and that these have not been met, which may be a very painful and sad realisation that we've been avoiding.

If we're very deeply caught in one of these patterns, we may benefit from specialised therapeutic help. But we can also explore working with these issues through the Alexander Technique. Suppose we tend to inhabit the collapsed, hopeless-feeling end of the continuum. In that case our teacher will hopefully gently encourage us to become aware of *glimmers*—little moments of ease, glimpses of wholeness and lightness, warmth and human contact, no matter how small they may be. Gradually, if we persist, we may see that although so much that was needed was missing in the past, there is goodness still to be found in the present.

On the physical level we may look at finding our way gently out of our collapsed slump, gradually discovering that there's the possibility of support from the Earth beneath us, and natural, spontaneous support to be found in our back and spine if only we allow it. What a revelation! Even if we weren't supported as we should've been by others in the past, we can find support now *in ourselves*. We discover we can choose, quite literally, not to be down but to be up. The accompanying change in how we feel about ourselves and the world around us may be as profound as the change in the way we physically look and feel.

If we tend to be more of a helper, on the other hand, our lessons and practice can become a place where we put ourselves first. To begin with, this can feel strange and uncomfortable. But perhaps, in time, we can let go of our set jaw and discover a bit of lightness and ease in our body and our over-helping hands and feet. We can learn to say no to the impulse to rush to put others first, taking time to breathe, settle, and come back to ourselves, to our bodies and to our own true needs.

Difficulties With Expression and Trust

As well as having our physical needs met, as young children we also need to be seen, validated, and given the message that we're basically OK by those around us. This becomes particularly important as we start to discover that we have feelings about things and that we want to express them to others. We need to know that, even if people don't always agree with us, we have a right to feel what we feel and that these feelings will be taken seriously. If this early acceptance and validation are lacking, it can lead to deep feelings of shame and unworthiness based on the sense that the essence of who we are isn't acceptable to those around us.

This can have various outcomes. We may unconsciously decide that since showing our true selves seems to result in rejection and pain, it's better not to be seen at all. In later life, we may avoid expressing ourselves, hiding who we really are. At the same time, we may feel misunderstood and angry that our true self is apparently not wanted. Because we don't trust others to accept our feelings and needs if we express them openly and straightforwardly, we may become quite skilled at getting what we want in more subtle ways. We may become adept at manipulating people and situations, exercising considerable power from behind what seems, on the surface, to be a modest, unassuming demeanour.

A more troubling outcome may be that we project our feelings of unworthiness outwards. It's not *us* that's the problem, it's those others! Rather than experiencing the shame of not being acceptable, we put it onto other people, putting them down in our minds so that we can feel superior. To maintain this elevated self-image we will need to gain acclaim and approval—not by showing our true selves, which we are ashamed of, but by presenting an impressive 'false self' for everyone to admire.

This is what we call narcissism, and in its more extreme forms it can be very difficult to be around because such a person doesn't feel much empathy and is often happy to trample on others to gain the validation they crave. They may tend to puff their chest out in an expression of superiority, though their heart remains closed. Or they may adopt some other characteristic posture that openly or covertly projects a sense of superiority and entitlement.

Their smile may be more of a smirk as they contemplate the inferiority of those around them.

If we have these kinds of shame-based wounds it can interfere in various ways with learning a practice like the Alexander Technique. For a start, we're likely to be holding a lot of muscular tension around our chest as we puff ourselves up or try to protect our heart from being hurt again. This holding and tension can get in the way of the natural, free movements of the breath. In addition, we may disconnect from our bodily sensations because it's through the body that we experience our true feelings, including ones of vulnerability which we find uncomfortable and shameful. We may find refuge in rationalisation, thinking at the expense of feeling, cutting ourselves off from the vital information our body offers us from moment to moment. And because shame is such a painful emotion, the fear of experiencing it can make it particularly difficult to let go of these patterns.

But perhaps, if our teacher is sensitive to such things, Alexander lessons can be a place where we can gradually discover, in a very tangible, embodied way, that we can show ourselves and make gestures, sounds, and shapes that reflect who we are without being shamed. Perhaps we can allow ourselves to begin to notice our bodily sensations, to trust a little more, and to let the area around our heart open so that we can be seen. In time, this may open the door to us being able to be more straightforward in our interactions with others, so that we can get what we need from them in a more direct and healthy way.

If we're the sort of person who has been inclined to turn our shame outwards, though, there's a good chance we won't come for lessons or therapy in the first place.

What could *we* possibly have to learn from *them* anyway? But maybe we reach a point where there's a crack in our armour. Something's gone wrong once too often. We notice that life isn't going well and that we're increasingly lonely. We realise we could use a little help. If so, perhaps we can very slowly and gently allow the tightness around our heart to loosen and open. We can let go of postures that project self-importance and land fully on the ground rather than pulling ourselves up and away to be above it all. Perhaps we can begin to face some of the shame we've been hiding behind our false self and gradually let ourselves arrive with the others on planet Earth. Things will be very different from then on.

Difficulties With Releasing and Letting Go

When we're still very young, there comes a time when we need to begin to gain a sense of independence and self-determination. In particular, we need to begin to take responsibility for our own bodies and needs. We need to notice when we're hungry, sleepy, or need the toilet, or when we want to be serious, laugh, or dance about, and we need to learn to give those impulses permission in an appropriate way.

But what if our carers have trouble letting go of their control over us? What if they're anxious themselves and express that anxiousness by seeking to maintain control of our actions and bodies beyond a point that's helpful?

Excessive control from caregivers can appear in various ways, causing us to get into the habit of forcefully pushing down, restraining, and holding onto our natural, healthy impulses. Eating or not eating, relieving ourselves, expressing our thoughts and opinions, how we spend our time, balancing work and leisure—these areas and others can all be affected by excessive external control.

Of course we do need to control our natural impulses sometimes or there would be chaos, but healthy control comes from *within*. It's not forced from outside but arises from a grounded, open-hearted wish to participate in society productively, but on our own terms.

Holding back our healthy impulses is a very embodied thing. We *literally* hold on with our muscles. When these compulsive holding patterns develop at a young age it can lead to patterns of unconscious bracing throughout the body and great difficulty in allowing things in and around us to flow freely. This will be an issue if we're doing a practice like the Alexander Technique which relies on us being willing to let go of control so that natural processes and movements can manifest and express. After all, this was precisely the freedom that was banned so many years ago.

Letting go of this deeply embedded bracing may, for some people, evoke feelings of anger and shame that are locked up within it. It can take some courage—and a patient teacher, or perhaps the help of a skilled therapist— to give those feelings and that compulsive holding permission to let go.

One thing that can be particularly helpful if we're a 'holding' sort of character is dancing. Not the sort of formal, structured dancing that has steps to learn, but the free, improvisational, expressive dancing you can experience in group dance practices like 5Rhythms, Biodanza, and Dance of Awareness. If you try one of these you may find to begin with that your tendency to hold on and resist your body's natural impulses keeps throwing you out of the rhythm. But in time the compelling pulse of the music and of the other dancers may be enough to encourage you through the resistance, carrying you along with it, allowing you to let go at last and release into the flow.

The Process of Change

Of course, the character traits I've been describing in this chapter are caricatures to some extent. It would be a mistake to take any of them completely literally as portraits of ourselves or other people. But at the same time, there may well be at least *something* of yourself to be recognised in them. It's worth thinking about. Where might you be blocked? What factors might be standing in the way of *your* system's inherent tendency to be open and free, grounded, dynamic, and delicately breathing in movement and at rest?

The fact that a degree of psychophysical resolution and release is often needed to enable our system to really settle into ease underlines the need for patience in our practice. We may want to progress as quickly as possible but there are often very good reasons why it will take longer than we wish. There may need to be a process of emotional integration, a letting go of muscular armouring, and an accompanying process of making sense of ourselves and our lives in a new way. None of this can be rushed. Change and integration take as long as they take, no matter how much of a hurry we might be in. But if we give it time, gently, quietly, without stress and strain, we will get there. All this is part of the value of a practice like the Alexander Technique. It's not just the practice itself but what else it opens up for us—where it points to, what it suggests to us about who we are, where we've been, where we're going, and who we might one day become.

Chapter Thirty-Two
The Road Ahead

We think things are simple. Or we think they are merely complex.
— Tom Cheetham, Green Man, Earth Angel

Throughout this book I've written a lot about how you might change your state of being and the way you move and do things for the better—but possibly in a way that is rather different from what you were expecting when you first picked it up. Instead of giving step-by-step instructions, I've been circling the problem, going round and round various key ideas and concepts, looking at the parts of the puzzle from different perspectives: 'You can think about it this way . . . and you can think about it that way'. We've looked at things from an objective, science-like perspective and from an in-the-moment, experiential perspective. We've explored the Self from the angle of the body, the mind, the emotions and the interaction between them. We've explored how things are when they're going right and when they're going rather less right. We've thought about things in theory and we've begun to put them into practice.

Perhaps you've liked this open-ended, exploratory approach, but maybe, even now, you're finding it a little frustrating. Sometimes we don't want *this* way and *that* way—we want *the* way! In hoping to change the Self, however, we're dealing with a dynamic whole made up of many interrelated and interacting parts, and one of those parts is the personal, voluntary self that is seeking to bring the change about. It's a complex situation. There's no simple, foolproof, step-by-step formula we can apply to this intricate being. But through circling, exploring, thinking and experimenting, in time our understanding develops and grows. Rather than being simple or 'merely complex' it becomes *deep*. More and more we find we can be in the activity of our lives and at the same time stepping back, seeing what needs to happen and what we must do and not do from moment to moment to allow ease and skilfulness to manifest.

The principles we've been exploring in this book can enable you to change in ways that may surprise you and can make a significant difference in your life. They can lead to experiences which are genuinely transformative and new, which aren't just the same-old-same-old dressed up in a different way. Principles, you see, can be powerful things. Say for example that we accept the principle that taking a sensible amount of exercise is good for us. We're none the wiser about whether it would be best to go for a walk, run or swim, row a boat or go rock climbing. But the principle still guides us towards getting up off the sofa and raising a sweat in one way or another. We could do some conventional form of exercise or even invent an entirely new one and we'd still be honouring the principle. And while the principle tells us we should do some exercise (a 'sensible amount'), it leaves us free to determine how much that might be in the context of our particular lives and goals. Principles both guide and leave us free *at the same time*.

Similarly, the principles underlying ease and skilfulness don't define precisely what to do and how to do it. They don't give us a rigid template. They're propositions about the way things work. Used wisely they can act as a yardstick to guide us towards sensible, intelligent, creative choices of our own. Rather than pushing us along rigidly predetermined channels they keep our options open while at the same time guiding our choices towards actions that are wise, healthy and free.

Before we finish, I want to leave you with a couple of final thoughts. You might have noticed that there's a word in this book that I've used over and over again. It's not a technical word but one that denotes a quality, and that word is 'gently'.

A common belief around learning and growing is that it will be—or even should be—hard work. We may feel that we'll need to discipline ourselves and try really hard at it. Many of us admire a person who drives themselves to various forms of success, and feel that by applying maximum effort we, too, will get the results we want.

Of course we do need to apply ourselves to things in life and bring some commitment and focus to our attempts to learn and change. But at the same time, these good intentions can have a shadow side. If they're taken to excess we can become rather *unkind* to ourselves. We can start to take it all too seriously and get quite judgemental about ourselves and our speed of progress. We may be so keen to get the results we want (particularly if we're in pain or suffering in some way and hoping for relief) that we become a bit obsessive about it all, never letting go and just living, creating a false distance between ourselves and our life. So if you decide to explore the suggestions in this book, I hope you'll bear this in mind and be kind and gentle with yourself, as much as you are able.

Another way of talking about this is to say that no matter how much we want to get to where we're going, we also need to nurture pleasure in the journey. Imagine walking the great Camino to Santiago. You'd probably find that the rewards weren't so much in reaching the end as they were in being on the road itself, step by step, day by day—in the rhythm of moving through a great landscape, through chance meetings, fellowship and challenges.

Sometimes we sacrifice all the pleasure of the road in our hurry to be at our destination. We're like someone walking the Camino with their head down, determined to arrive first. What a waste! But at the same time we mustn't let go of all intention, focus and direction—wandering off the track all the time, getting lost, constantly sitting down by the roadside and falling asleep, talking to every passerby whether they want to talk with us or not. The summer ends and we never even reached Santiago.

'Don't care anyway,' we say.

But perhaps we do really, deep down.

But what if, instead of being in conflict, these two perspectives can come into a rich dialogue with each other? What if they can complement each other rather than being opposed? What if the journey can be enriching, a pleasure in itself, while still ending in a triumphant arrival? Because finding true ease and skilfulness is neither a gung-ho pursuit nor an abandonment of purpose and direction. Rather it's a delicate dance between different perspectives. It's not an argument or a competition: it's a *conversation*.

And so, with that, we have reached the end of our journey and perhaps the beginning of another one. If you came to this book with some experience of Alexander work, I hope that you've gained a few new ideas or ways of looking at things that will be helpful. And if this has all been new to you, I hope some of the things I've said have been intriguing enough to make you want to explore further, and that you'll feel free to begin doing so right now, on your own. But at the same time, on a journey through unfamiliar terrain it can be good to have a guide to walk with you for a while: someone who already knows the territory, who can help you avoid the pitfalls and take you to interesting places that you might never find without them. Do think about finding yourself a teacher! This work is rich and interesting. For over a century it has attracted thoughtful and interesting people who have each been on their own journey with it and come to see it in their own way. So why not find someone to show you? Someone you like, who seems open-minded and curious, who isn't in a hurry and who has something interesting to say about it all. I expect you'll find it will be worth your while.

Appendices

Appendix A
Note For Alexander Teachers

Don't be surprised, Socrates, if amid so many opinions we can't find explanations that are completely consistent with one another! Instead, be satisfied if we come up with stories that are as likely as any others—after all, we are only mortal men.
—PLATO, Timaeus

In the Preface I described the origins of some of the various threads that have come together in this book, but the decision to actually sit down and write it came from a sense of frustration which was essentially about concepts and jargon. There are lots of good books about the Alexander Technique, and I often suggest to my students that they read one or other of them in the hope it will get them thinking about themselves and the way their minds and bodies function. But all too often they'll come back and, instead, ask questions about the meaning of words.

'What is "direction"?'

'What is "the primary control"?'

'What is "inhibition"?'

And then, before you know it, we're talking about these jargon terms and what they 'really mean', which, though not uninteresting, seems to me to be missing the point. Because what I'm actually hoping for is to be having discussions with them about how their body and nervous system work, encouraging them to understand as deeply as possible why their system is not functioning as well as it might and what could improve things, so that these understandings naturally lead to them making more healthy, harmonious choices.

As is quite common, my own early experience of learning the Alexander Technique, and of training to teach it, was both wonderful and frustrating. The wonderful part was often to do with having lovely experiences through some excellent hands-on work. The frustrating part was struggling for a long time to integrate and understand these experiences and make them my own.

Also around this time I'd begun exploring some more therapeutically based movement and embodiment practices which were giving me compelling but quite different experiences of being in a body. Increasingly I was wanting to find a conception of the work that was broad and rich enough to remain true to itself while being able to comfortably encompass these other interesting things I was discovering.

Among all this, I'd been coming into contact with outlier Alexander teachers whose conceptions didn't quite fit within the established model as it appears in F.M.'s books. It was beginning to feel as if life and human functioning were turning out to be too wide and rich to fully fit within the traditional bounds of the Technique so that they kept bursting out around the edges.

So, like many other simultaneously enthusiastic and questioning Alexander teachers have done before and since, I decided to start over, beginning as much as possible from what I could observe in myself and working outwards rather than starting with the established tradition with its jargon words, concepts and practices and trying to work my way back *in* from there. I trusted that, in so far as the things that F.M. was pointing to were valid, I would come across them in my own time and way.

Doing this is an interesting endeavour, because if we

start looking at something from where we are, rather than from where someone else *was*, we'll inevitably be bringing our own background, quirks and context to it, and so are bound to end up viewing the same things in a slightly different way. This is particularly true when looking at ourselves and our functioning, which we can't help but view subjectively, conditioned by our experiences, cultural context and assumptions. We can never get to a conclusive truth about the way things are or about how we or others should best address our challenges and difficulties. The most we can hope to come up with is, as Plato puts it, a 'likely story' which is *true enough* to be worth the telling.

Influences

Many people and ideas have influenced this book apart from F.M. Alexander and my various teachers. One of the most formative was Fiona Robb's little book, *Not to 'Do'*, which recounts her lessons with Margaret Goldie in the 1990s. I never met Miss Goldie, but somehow Robb's portrayal of her dogged insistence on not doing made things land for me in a way that nothing or no one else had quite managed until then. This growing understanding eventually merged with a pre-existing interest in mysticism and neti-neti to produce the not-this-not-that approach outlined in this book.

Also around this time I came into contact with David Gorman's radical pre-LearningMethods work which got me thinking about vicious circles ('The rounder we go the stucker we get'!) and caused me to further question the traditional view of the primary control which I was already feeling a little uncomfortable with. David's idea that support and balance are activated and organised primarily in relation to our attention and contact with the world around us was transformational for me at that time.

Another important influence was the late Chris Stevens. Chris was a scientist as well as an Alexander teacher, and he thought about balance, stabilisation and support differently to the more top-down way I had been familiar with. He would come into our training course in the 1990s and show us how getting out of the way of the equilibrium responses was an essential prerequisite to freedom and ease elsewhere. I vividly remember one astonishing 'turn' with him which literally flipped my understanding of how things work on its head.

Coming across Theodore Dimon's work, particularly his 2003 book *The Elements of Skill*, got me thinking more deeply about skilfulness, helping me to begin filling in some gaps in F.M.'s original formulation. Another book that encouraged me to think about some Alexander concepts from a different perspective was *Alexander Revisited* by Ron Dennis. Also, although I haven't had much direct contact with the predominantly US-based Marjorie Barstow tradition, I'm sure that, over the years, this more active, movement-based approach has influenced me through things I've come across that have washed up on these shores from across the Atlantic.

Much more recently, in 2016, I had the good fortune to attend a workshop run by Patrick Johnson and Tim Cacciatore in which they presented their work on the science of the Alexander Technique. The information they shared caused me to reassess several understandings I had absorbed over the years and made thinking about, teaching and explaining the Technique a lot more straightforward. Some of this material has ended up (filtered through my own understanding and presented in a more colloquial way) in the model of functioning described in Part One of the book.

As for the seven qualities of ease and the four characteristics of skilful action, these are distilled from observations that are common currency, shared not just with many Alexander teachers but with other mind–body disciplines as well. Many yoga and tai chi teachers, dancers, embodied therapists and somatic and embodiment practitioners would recognise them, or something very like them. But, at the same time, there's nothing set in stone about the particular qualities and characteristics I've chosen. I believe they offer a helpful way of getting a handle on ease and skilfulness, providing sufficient depth and enough angles from which to look at things without being overwhelming. But they're not definitive or exhaustive. There are other ways I could have divided up the pie, other qualities and characteristics I could have brought in, and other words I could have used to point towards the phenomena I've been describing.

Beyond the Alexander Technique, I've also been drawn to phenomenological writers such as Martin Heidegger, Maurice Merleau-Ponty and Hubert Dreyfus. Their approach is helpful in so far as they seek to describe and take seriously our embodied experience and meaning-making, focusing on how our bodies and actions are experienced at a subjective and relational level and taking that lived experience as the primary reality. An appreciation of this viewpoint, and the creative tension between it and more science-like, objective understandings, is an implicit theme of this book.

Another influence comes from a youthful interest in the teachings of Jiddu Krishnamurti. Although this interest waned, his recognition that seeing and understanding something deeply is inseparable from the wise action that arises from that seeing and understanding had a big impact. This has found its way particularly into Chapters Twenty-Three and Twenty-Five.

Finally, my approach has been influenced by my psychotherapy work and training. The model of trauma and the material around primitive defensive responses draws on Peter Levine and Babette Rothschild's work, and on polyvagal theory which, although increasingly seen as scientifically questionable, remains useful as a practical model for how anxiety and trauma manifest in the mind and body.

The neo-Reichian material has been influenced by Nick Totton and Laurence Heller's writings, and particularly by Tim Brown's work and by his help and mentorship as I ventured into the world of body-based therapy. His 'Body-listening' approach offers a gentler, more person-centred and process-oriented way into Reich's thinking than Reich's much more forceful way of working.

I have also benefitted from Brigitta Mowat's work on the intersection of therapy and the Alexander Technique which helped clarify my thinking when I started to realise that keeping the two worlds as far apart as they've traditionally been held no longer felt congruent, and was not always fully serving of my students' needs.

What About Direction?

Something that some Alexander teachers reading this book may be wondering about is 'direction'. How has such an important concept apparently gone missing? Perhaps it's still there in a sense, though.

As with several other Alexander Technique concepts, there are different views about what directing is and how it works. One way of thinking about it is that it gives us a clear image of what would be good for us. This acts like a mirror, helping us to notice whatever we're up to which *isn't* that so we can choose not to do it. If I think about my neck being free, for example, this encourages me to notice anything I'm up to that is causing it to tighten. From this perspective, direction can be seen as a guiding framework that helps us to make sensible negative choices.

In a sense, the qualities of ease I've suggested in this book are very similar to directions because, like them, they represent the positive side of the equation. They're the things that we *want*. But rather than making the thinking about those things into a discrete 'thing' in itself, or a skill to learn and apply, I'm suggesting that we simply bring a natural curiosity and interest about these qualities to ourselves and our situation.

If you're walking along and you see a hole in the road, you don't deliberately project a mental image of how to get past it that's in any sense separate from your dealing with the problem in the normal way of things. Having seen the hole and realised the implications, you just step around it. Your understanding of the situation leads to sensible action without a separate procedure needing to be inserted between that situation and yourself.

Similarly, if we're interested and curious about the way our system works and what we're up to from moment to moment, there's no need for directing in the sense of deliberately thinking, wishing or asking for what we want as an act that is in any way apart from that. A straightforward, practical appreciation of what's needed and not needed arises from our curiosity, interest and growing understanding, naturally and unforcedly, on its own.

While your mileage may vary, this seems to me to be a pleasingly simple way of going about things. It also avoids some of the common difficulties around inadvertently trying to *do* the directions which people frequently get caught in (often even after many years of practice) and that can sometimes—particularly if a student is prone to anxiety and over-doing—cause real harm.

Appendix B
When the Right Thing *Can't* Do Itself

Alexander teachers make quite a bold claim, which I've repeated throughout this book, which is that if we would only get out of the way of our body's spontaneous mechanisms our system will self-organise in a free and easy way. This is generally true, but there's also a problem with the argument which is that it assumes the underlying spontaneous systems are working as they should be. Generally they are, because they're quite robust, but for some people, for various reasons, they are not. Factors like injury or certain health conditions—particularly those which interfere with the functioning of the nervous system such as cerebral palsy, Parkinson's, multiple sclerosis or strokes—can leave our system compromised and unable to organise with dynamic ease even if we're able to get out of its way.

However, this doesn't mean that the ideas in this book will be ineffective. For a start, our spontaneous systems are never *totally* compromised. Where they don't work as well as they might we have to take up the slack with increased voluntary control. But that control needs to be appropriate, and no more intrusive or over-effortful than it absolutely has to be, allowing our spontaneous functions to play their role where they are able while gently filling in the gaps where they are not.

The principles in this book are well suited to helping with this. It's still just as good for us to be as present, quiet, open and free as possible, and to be moving with as much ease and skill as we can—and the qualities of ease and the characteristics of skilful action can still function as help-ful guides towards doing so. We can still be wondering whether what we're up to is congruent with those qualities and characteristics, and about what may be interfering or getting in the way of them. And while giving voluntary support to our system, we can still choose not to do any-thing that isn't absolutely necessary. The principles work in the same way, and can be a valuable resource in helping us to find as much ease and skilfulness as possible in the circumstances we find ourselves in.

Retained Primitive Reflexes

One phenomenon which can interfere with our system's ability to healthily self-organise is retained primitive reflexes. Primitive reflexes are automatic reflex responses that babies are born with (such as the sucking reflex, the infant startle (Moro) reflex and various others) which automatically coordinate movements and responses that are essential for a newborn baby's survival. Generally these reflexes disappear in the first six months or so of life, to be gradually replaced by more mature ones and the volun-tary movement patterns the child will need as an adult. But sometimes they persist, interfering unhelpfully with our mature reflex and voluntary movement systems. This can contribute to problems with coordination, balance, sensory perception, fine motor skills, impulse control, focus and social and academic learning. It can also interfere with learning a practice like the Alexander Technique, because the retained primitive reflex responses may be constantly getting triggered, needing to be voluntarily suppressed with muscular tension or getting in the way of the body's attempts to organise spontaneous dynamic stabilisation, balance and support.

Fortunately it's possible to integrate retained primitive reflexes later in life. Various programmes have been developed to test for their presence and to resolve any that are found. You can find further resources in the reading list in Appendix D.

Appendix C
Regulating Anxiety States

We've seen throughout this book that anxiety is one of the biggest barriers to experiencing more ease and skilfulness in our lives. Even the most calm and grounded of us can get overwhelmed by anxiety now and again, so we can all use a bit of help to enable us to calm down and regulate our nervous systems from time to time.

This is particularly important if we've been affected by trauma, leaving us with very strong and easily triggered anxiety responses. Knowing how to calm our nervous system when it's over-aroused can be particularly useful in such circumstances, and is also a helpful step towards resolving the underlying causes of the trauma.

Suppose a person who is chronically anxious comes for Alexander lessons. Initially it may be difficult or impossible for them to take even the first step of coming to a free and easy state of quiet, alert, open awareness. Their nervous system doesn't accept that the world is safe enough to let go and trust to that extent. They may need a lot of support to help their system to regulate and settle. If the anxiety is severe, this may be the main focus of the lessons for a long time, because until there is a degree of safety, everything else will remain jammed up by the ongoing anxiousness in their system.

We saw in Chapter Four that our primitive anxiety responses take one of three forms. There are fight–flight states (hyper-arousal), collapsed flop states (hypo-arousal) and frozen states which contain elements of both. Below are some suggestions for helping to regulate each of these states and to come back to calmness and balance. You'll find further ideas and information in some of the books about trauma listed in Appendix D. If the ideas here aren't helpful, or even seem to intensify your anxiousness—or if your anxiety is notably disruptive to your life or feels overwhelming—you should consider seeking professional help to learn to regulate your anxiety effectively and resolve any underlying causes.

Hyper-Arousal: Fight and Flight

Hyper-arousal comes from the high-energy, fight–flight parts of our primitive survival responses in which energy is aroused for self-defence. A person who tends towards these kinds of states may be on almost permanent high alert—always tense and easily startled, unable to settle, relax and enjoy life.

If you tend towards hyper-arousal, here are some things you can try which, with practice, may help you regulate your system and make you feel safer. If anything on the list doesn't feel helpful, it's fine to leave it and try some of the other ones instead:

- Look around you and listen to the sounds in your environment. This is a calming strategy that all creatures use. It can help to give your nervous system the confidence that—at least in this moment—you know where you are and that you're physically safe.

- Notice bodily sensations such as your breathing, feelings of movement, temperature, the texture of your clothes and the surface of your skin, allowing your attention to move freely from place to place.

- Bring attention to your out breath. This tends to activate the calming action of the parasympathetic nervous system. Try lengthening your out-breaths for a while to emphasise this calming effect.

• Have a few gentle sighs or a good yawn. These are natural ways of releasing nervous tension common to all mammals.

• Try letting your body move, just as it feels inclined to.

• Notice where in your body feels stronger and more secure. No matter how anxious we feel there's almost always somewhere in us that has a slightly different point of view. When you find such a place, enjoy lightly resting your attention there for a while.

• Pay attention to 'glimmers'. Glimmers are moments when we have a feeling (no matter how small or short-lived) of ease, contentment or happiness. Sometimes we may get so caught up in our worries about what's wrong that we don't notice the things that are OK, depriving our nervous system of the feeling of safety and security that these experiences provide.

• Remember a specific incident from the past where you felt safe, happy, strong, nurtured or content. Close your eyes and mentally put yourself back there remembering in detail the sights, sounds, smells and how it felt in your body (this is called anchoring).

• Notice the feeling of support that comes from the ground beneath you or from any surface you're sitting or lying on or against.

• Make contact with yourself, perhaps placing your hands on your heart and belly or anywhere else that you're drawn to, consciously telling your body through the quality of your touch, 'It's OK, you are safe!'

• Try singing or humming to yourself. Gentle use of the voice tends to activate the parasympathetic nervous system, helping to you to calm down.

• If there's a calm, trusted person available, try reaching out to them. Their calmness is likely to be infectious.

None of these is an instant cure for an anxious, over-stimulated nervous system. But if when you feel anxious you take time to play around with some of the ones that appeal to you, you may gradually start to notice the effects. These may be subtle to begin with, but in time they join up to give you a real, tacit understanding of how to regulate your emotional state and calm yourself down.

Hyper/Hypo-Arousal: Freeze

Hyper-aroused states have a feeling of energy and movement about them. When we're in more frozen states, on the other hand, our system is still anxiously aroused but we find it difficult to move and take action. We may have a feeling of restless anxiousness or even dread while feeling simultaneously somewhat helpless and stuck.

This sense of anxious immobility may be very strong or quite mild, but in its origins it's similar to the response of a mouse frozen in front of a cat. All the mouse's energy is aroused for fight or flight, but its parasympathetic nervous system is 'putting on the brakes' because its limbic brain has decided it's safest not to move. The moment there's the slightest opening, though, the mouse will burst into action again using all that pent-up energy to escape.

Some of the techniques I suggested for hyper-arousal can also help us shift out of frozen states too, particularly those which activate us and draw us out of ourselves, such as gently moving our body, looking around us and focusing awareness on our environment. Connecting with other people can also be very helpful. Techniques that take our awareness inwards, such as focusing on our physical sensations, thoughts or memories, are likely to be less helpful, because in frozen states our attention tends to be directed excessively inwards already.

Just like the mouse, when we come out of a frozen state we'll tend to come into a more mobilised, high-energy state as the parasympathetic brake is taken off. The strength of this response can take us by surprise, and even alarm us if we're not used to it. However, from that more hyper-activated place we then have a chance to apply regulating techniques to bring ourselves gently back to balance.

Hypo-Arousal: Flop

So far I've been talking about anxiety states that have some energy about them, even if that energy is frozen. Sometimes, however—particularly if a person has been in threatening situations in which there seemed to be no way out and there was no friendly voice or face to help—their system may tend towards states of hypo-arousal instead. The shutdown state of hypo-arousal is the most basic line of defence that our system goes to when hope seems lost. It is associated with the 'flop' part of our primitive survival responses, making us feel to a greater or lesser degree heavy, withdrawn, inward-looking, depressed and immobilised, or causing us to experience dissociated states where it feels as if we're not quite in our body.

As with the other states we've been considering, hypo-arousal can be relatively mild or very deep. If we tend towards these kinds of shutdown, collapsed, depressed states and they're not too deep, we may be able to shift out of them on our own by gently activating in various ways. For example:

- We can gently lengthen and deepen both our in-breath and our out-breath. The longer in-breath encourages our sympathetic nervous system to activate to help nudge us out of collapse towards a more energised state.

- As with frozen states, we can see if we can bring our attention gently out of ourselves, noticing particularly what we can touch, see and hear in the world around us.

- We can begin to gently move our bodies.

- We can do creative, tactile, artistic activities such as drawing, painting or sculpting.

- We can put on some gentle music and move to it, or try humming, singing or playing a musical instrument.

Similar to when we move out of a frozen state, moving out of hypo-arousal may be accompanied by a surge of energy as our sympathetic nervous system re-activates, and from that more active state we can then apply calming strategies to help our system settle and return to balance. For some people, though, this shift into hyper-arousal can be so strong that it feels frightening enough to send them straight back into hypo-arousal again!

If this see-sawing between hypo- and hyper-arousal is familiar to you, or it feels like the simple suggestions above are too much or are ineffective at the moment or you feel overwhelmed, you should think about finding some professional assistance to help you learn how to regulate your nervous system in a safe, contained way and to address whatever past events caused you to be prone to these states in the first place.

Appendix D
Further Reading

If you want to get a sense of where the ideas and approach in this book come from, and of some different ways people have thought about the Alexander Technique over the years, here are some resources for you to explore.

The obvious place to start is with the books of F.M. Alexander himself. There are a couple of things to be aware of, though. The first is that his old-fashioned writing style can be heavy going for some modern readers. The second is that, unfortunately, there is some unpleasant racism in some of his discussions about wider issues that appear alongside his transformational insights into human functioning.

However, the practice and theory of the Alexander Technique aren't dependent on or defined by these elements in his writing, and there is one very readable book which largely avoids them. It's called *The Use of the Self* and it is still in print today. If you'd like to try another of his books, *Constructive Conscious Control of the Individual* is a good second choice, while to get a concise taste of his thinking about the Technique, his *Aphorisms* are published by the specialist Alexander Technique publisher Mouritz.

There have been many other books written about the Technique apart from Alexander's own. Some good introductory ones are: *A Skill for Life*, by Pedro de Alcantara; *How You Stand, How You Move, How You Live* by Missy Vineyard; *Principles of the Alexander Technique* by Jeremy Chance; and *Finding Quiet Strength* by Judith Kleinman.

An older book worth looking at is *Freedom to Change* by Frank Pierce Jones.

If you want to look beyond the basics, some other writings which have particularly influenced the approach in this book are *Not to 'Do'* by Fiona Robb; *Looking at Ourselves* by David Gorman; *The Elements of Skill* by Theodore Dimon; *Alexander Revisited* by Ron Dennis; and *The Act of Living* by Walter Carrington.

If you'd like a book that explores a more heart-centred way of working with Alexander Technique principles you may enjoy *Teaching by Hand, Learning by Heart* by Bruce Fertman.

There's some useful information about body mapping in *What Every Musician Needs to Know About the Body* by Barbara Conable, and also in *How to Learn the Alexander Technique* by William and Barbara Conable.

Many musicians are drawn to the Alexander Technique. A good place for them to start is another book by Pedro de Alcantara called *Indirect Procedures*.

Finally, if you want to explore some of the science that has been done around the Alexander Technique, you could begin with a paper by Timothy W. Cacciatore, Patrick M. Johnson and Rajal G. Cohen called 'Potential Mechanisms of the Alexander Technique: Toward a Comprehensive Neurophysiological Model', published in 2020 in the *Kinesiology Review*, Volume 9: Issue 3.

Beyond the Alexander Technique

A helpful introduction to Reichian theory and practice can be found in Nick Totton and Em Edmondson's book, *Reichian Growth Work*. You could also go straight to the source and look at *Character Analysis* by Wilhelm Reich or

The Language of the Body by Alexander Lowen, one of Reich's early disciples. A more recent reworking of Reich's character structures model can be found in Laurence Heller's *Healing Developmental Trauma*.

A good practical source for information about anxiety, trauma and emotional regulation is Deb Dana's *Anchored*, which is based on polyvagal theory. Peter Levine's *In an Unspoken Voice* and Babette Rothschild's *The Body Remembers* are good on trauma, arousal and primitive defence responses.

Finally, if you're interested in following up on the information in Appendix B about retained primitive reflexes, you could begin with Sally Goddard's book *Reflexes, Learning and Behaviour, a Window into the Child's Mind*.

Index

A

acting (performance arts) 221

action sequences 80–83, 85–87, 146.
See also sequences (of
movements).
'unhealthy' action sequences 82–
83, 85

adrenaline 26

Alexander, Frederick Mattias xiv,
xxii, 11, 13, 16, 132, 167

alignment 39, 123, 132–133, 153, 163,
200

all fours 55, 58, 71, 105, 198–199, 202

allowing 168–170, 220, 222

anger 25–26, 129–130, 205

animals 5–8, 25, 27, 29, 32, 42, 66,
71–73, 104, 106, 113, 127, 129, 193,
206
dogs 32, 71, 104

anxiety 23, 74, 100, 120–123, 162, 252

appendicular skeleton. See skeleton,
axial and appendicular skeleton.

armouring 131. See also Reich,
Wilhelm.

arteries 18–19

atlanto-occipital joint. See skeleton,
atlanto-occipital joint.

attention 31, 34–37, 73, 81, 95, 98,
100, 123, 157

attunement 214–215. See also non-
verbal communication.

axial skeleton. See skeleton, axial
and appendicular skeleton.

B

balance 58–64, 132

base of support 58–63, 112–113, 188,
200

biceps. See muscles, biceps and triceps.

bicycle 11, 77

blood flow 17–18, 206

body mapping 135, 191, 265

body weight 54–55, 111, 115, 180, 183,
187
bracing caused by 111

Bodylistening 252

boundaries 216

bracing 39–42, 56, 180, 183–184, 187
pre-emptive 184–185
spontaneous 42, 103, 111

breathing 18–20, 22–23, 101
bucket handle 22–23, 102
high-arousal 24
low-arousal 20
pump handle 23–24

Brown, Tim 228, 252

busyness 122, 149, 194, 219

C

Cacciatore, Tim 265

capillaries 18

central pattern generators 67, 114

centre of gravity 55, 58, 63. See also
centred.

centred 60. See also centredness
(state of ease).

centredness (state of ease) 102, 109,
112, 156, 188

cerebral palsy 255

cervical spine. See skeleton, spine,
cervical.

characteristics of skilful action 108,
188

choice 12, 83–85, 87, 138, 146
negative choices 165, 175

circling the problem 86, 176, 193

competence 10

Conable, Barbara 265

Conable, William 265
concentration 34–37, 42, 125–126
    spontaneous versus voluntary 35
contact 211–213
coordination 65–66, 114
craniosacral therapy 231

D

Dana, Deb 266
dancing 72, 203, 215, 220–221
    conscious dance 220
deep muscles. *See* muscles, deep.
Dennis, Ron 250, 265
desk work 128
diaphragm. *See* muscles, diaphragm.
digestion 17–20, 26, 28–29
Dimon, Theodore 250
direction (Alexander Technique
    concept of) 252
dissociation 216
driving 82, 84, 87

E

economy 113
Edmondson, Em 265
effort 4, 110–111, 113–114, 132–133
emotions 25, 28–30, 74–75, 80–81,
    128–131, 205–207, 239, 266
endgaining 11, 117, 123, 153, 177
equilibrium responses 63, 250
explicit knowledge 77, 181. *See also*
    procedural understanding.
expression (artistic) 221
expression (emotional) 217–221
exteroceptive senses 31
eyes 32–36
    eye contact 75

F

feet 104–106, 112, 114, 116–117, 158,
    198, 202
field of attention 34–36
fight–flight response 26
floor 194–198
flop response 25, 27

flow (characteristic of skilful
    action) 116, 118, 150, 155, 188–189,
    192, 201
four buttons (metaphor) 169
freedom (quality of ease) 101–102
freeze response 25–27, 42, 121, 213

G

Goddard, Sally 266
Goldie, Margaret 249
Gorman, David 265
gravity 38–39, 41, 44, 54–55, 58, 60–
    64, 115, 132, 141
grounded support 104–107

H

habits 83–86, 149, 162, 177
head–neck joint. *See* skeleton,
    head–neck joint.
heart 18–19, 26, 28–29

I

implicit knowledge 77. *See also*
    procedural understanding.
inertia 61–62. *See also* momentum.
integration 109–110
intention 183
intercostal muscles. *See* muscles,
    intercostals.
intermediate muscles. *See* muscles,
    intermediate.
interoceptive senses 31

J

jargon 247–248
Johnson, Patrick 250

K

Kinghorn, Bill xi
Kleinman, Judith 264

L

laugh 102, 129, 206, 218, 221
learned fear responses 121–122

Levine, Peter xvi
likely story 249
limbic brain 19, 26, 28, 74, 121
limbs 51, 85
lived experience 251
low-arousal states 29
Lowen, Alexander 266
lumbar spine. *See* skeleton, spine, lumbar.
lunging 200
lungs 16, 18–21, 23

M

mind–body 14, 16, 251
momentum 61–62, 115–116. *See also* inertia.
motor programmes 66–67
movement 65, 114, 116–118, 133
Mowat, Brigitta 252
multiple sclerosis 255
muscles 39–41, 49, 51, 54–55, 57
    biceps and triceps 39–40
    deep 49–50, 55
    diaphragm 20–23, 101
    intercostals 20, 49
    intermediate 49, 55
    superficial 49, 55
    synergies 66–67, 114
music 196–197, 202–203, 215–217, 220
mysticism 249

N

neck 24, 36, 46, 48–49, 105
negation 172
neti-neti 172–173, 249. *See also* not-this-not-that.
non-verbal communication 215. *See also* attunement.
not doing 163, 165, 249
not-this-not-that 172–173, 214, 219–221. *See also* neti-neti.

O

objective understanding 76, 251
openness

as quality of ease 99–102
    in field of attention 34–36
ordering (sequence of movements) 116–117
orienting 33–35
    involuntary orienting response 33
    voluntary orienting response 33–34

P

parasympathetic nervous system 19, 29, 75
Parkinson's disease 255
patience 176, 189
pausing 155–156, 192–193, 200
pelvis. *See* skeleton, pelvis.
perception 31
performance arts 221
peripheral zone. *See* vision, peripheral zone.
Peter Levine 252, 266
phenomenology 251
polyvagal theory xvi
practising 143, 147–149
predators 27, 36, 206
presence 98–99, 147–148, 156
principles 240
procedural understanding 76–77, 79. *See also* explicit knowledge, implicit knowledge.
proprioceptive senses 31, 76, 99, 132, 183
psychotherapy xv–xvi, 206, 252

Q

qualities of ease 94, 96, 109, 156, 173
quasistatic motion 61
quietness (quality of ease) 96–98

R

recumbent positions 115, 196
reflexes 16, 63
Reich, Wilhelm xv, 131. *See also* armouring.
repression 128, 130–131, 137, 205–206
ribcage. *See* skeleton, ribcage.

righting reactions 63
Robb, Fiona 249
Rothschild, Babette xvi
rushing 123–124

S

sacrum. *See* skeleton, spine, sacrum.
sadness 102, 128–131, 205
saying no 166–167
science 15, 94, 239
Self 13–14
   spontaneous self 16
   voluntary self 15
   voluntary activity 15
self-defence 26, 92, 206
semi-supine position 194
sensing 31–35
sequences (of movements) 199–202.
   See also action sequences.
shaking 130, 206–207
shame 27
shapes (expressive) 217
shoulder girdle. *See* skeleton,
   shoulder girdle.
singing 101, 217, 219
sitting bones. *See* skeleton, sitting
   bones.
sitting up straight 126, 143, 165
skeleton
   atlanto-occipital joint 48
   axial and appendicular
   skeleton 44
   calcaneus 51
   carpals 51
   head–neck joint 48, 100–101, 105,
   134, 191
   hip joints 106, 110, 112, 134
   pelvis 44, 46, 51
   ribcage 20–22, 44–46, 49
   shoulder girdle
     collarbones 51
     shoulder blades 51, 53–54, 134
   sitting bones 51, 104
   skull 44, 48
   spine 44, 46, 48–49, 51, 55, 57
     atlanto-occipital joint 48

     cervical 46
     coccyx 46
     double curve 45
     lumbar 46, 134
     processes 46
     sacrum 46
     thoracic 46
     vertebrae 46
   tarsals 51
skilfulness 108–113, 116, 186, 188, 191,
   196, 198–199, 203
skilled pastimes 203
spine. *See* skeleton, spine.
squatting 199
stabilisation 38–39, 41–42
   braced stabilisation 39, 123, 183
   spontaneous stabilisation 41
standing (movement) 116, 153, 174,
   181, 186
standing (position) 104–105
stepping 67, 112, 114, 144
stopping doing 166
superficial muscles (of torso). *See*
   muscles, superficial.
support 44–46, 49, 51–52, 54–57
   braced support 56
   dynamic support 54, 105–107
survival energy 206–207
survival responses 25
sympathetic nervous system 19, 29
system (your system) 16

T

tacit understanding 78–79, 86
taking time 142–145
tangled thread (metaphor) 136–137,
   171
teachers 151–154
tears 16, 130, 206
thoracic spine. *See* skeleton, spine,
   thoracic.
tingling 206
torso 49, 51, 55, 57
tuning out 124

U

uncentred. *See* centred.
unfamiliar 149–150, 153, 163–164
unreliable sensory appreciation 132,
    156, 161, 163

V

vertebrae. *See* skeleton, spine,
    vertebrae.
vestibular sense 31
vicious circles 153
vision 32, 34–37, 64, 100
    central zone 34
    peripheral zone 34–35
voice 102, 211, 219, 221

W

washing the dishes 212
weight (balance) 59
weight (bodyweight). *See* body
    weight.
Whiteside, Abby xiii
whole self 14

Y

yawning 129, 142, 206